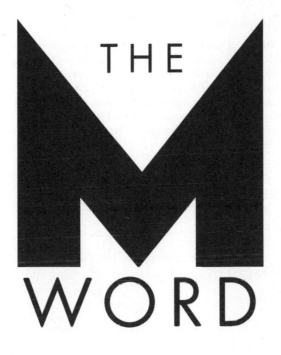

THE M WORD

Published in 2020 by Murdoch Books, an imprint of Allen & Unwin

Murdoch Books Australia
83 Alexander Street, Crows Nest NSW 2065
Phone: +61 (0)2 8425 0100
murdochbooks.com.au
info@murdochbooks.com.au

Murdoch Books UK
Ormond House, 26–27 Boswell Street, London WC1N 3JZ
Phone: +44 (0) 20 8785 5995
murdochbooks.co.uk
info@murdochbooks.co.uk

A catalogue record for this book is available from the British Library

ISBN 978 1 76052 487 6 Australia
ISBN 978 1 91163 238 2 UK

Cover design by Design By Committee
Text design by Susanne Geppert
Typeset by Midland Typesetters
Printed and bound in Great Britain by Clays Ltd, Elcograf S.p.A.

10 9 8

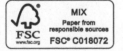

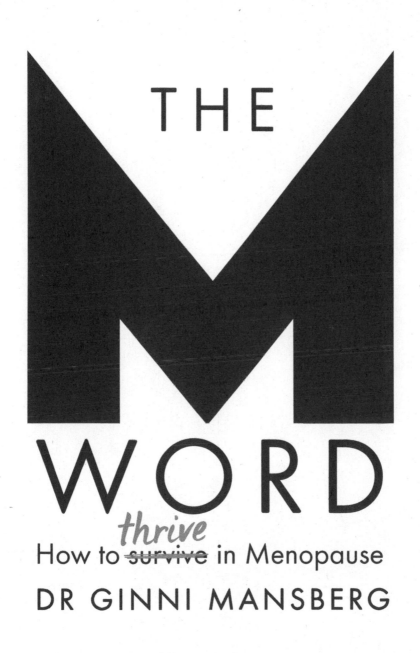

THE

M

WORD

How to ~~survive~~ *thrive* in Menopause

DR GINNI MANSBERG

murdoch books

Sydney | London

CONTENTS

INTRODUCTION

My nana used to call it the 'change of life'. It was a change alright. With menopause, many women like Nana went from feeling young and sexy to old almost overnight. Not only did they lose their periods and premenstrual tension (something that should have been an enormous relief), but many felt that they lost their femininity, too. With unpredictable hot sweats, grey pubic hair and dried-out vaginas, they often felt unattractive and useless. What possible value did they have? Besides caring for their elderly husbands and doing free babysitting for the grandchildren?

So when the 1980s rolled around and millions of women started taking the all-new hormone replacement therapy medication (HRT), the promised 'elixir of youth', things started looking up for menopausal women. Not only were they free of hot flushes (and remarkably free of wrinkles, too), but they were simultaneously riding high on a feminist revolution. This came courtesy of the trailblazers who had fought for their access to universities and career jobs, and the contraception that meant they didn't have to care for a dozen children. Plus the hairdressers who allowed them to banish grey hair, and the lawyers who got them out of marriages they didn't want to be in anymore. Not to mention the social security that meant being single wasn't a one-way ticket to the poor house.

Menopause meant finally letting go of the angst and self-doubt that had plagued them as younger women, and being ready to enjoy the next phase of their lives, a bit calmer, a bit sexier and a bit more financially secure than their mothers had been at the same stage.

But, as in all good stories, there was a twist. This is the tale of how one misguided press release, from a study claiming to be something it wasn't, triggered a feminist own-goal and saw the 'elixir of youth' rebranded as 'a potentially deadly beauty treatment' overnight. It was a moment that killed off a vital industry and led to an avalanche of suffering for millions of women.

The early termination, in 2002, of the Women's Health Initiative (WHI), a massive scientific study, was lauded in the media as a triumph of independent science over misogyny and the profiteering of drug companies from women's insecurities. The headlines blared that HRT was not the panacea for natural aging but instead, they claimed, it caused breast cancer. Overnight the use of HRT plummeted: women threw their pills in the bin; governments put out warnings; lawyers started suing; doctors refused to prescribe HRT and then lost the know-how to do it; and pharmaceutical companies rolled down the shutters on their women's health divisions.

So, women were told that hot flushes and painful vaginas weren't such terrible symptoms to endure. *Suck it up, Princess*, they were advised. Menopause Societies around the world tried to protest . . . *Stop. You've got it wrong. The WHI has been misinterpreted.* But their voices were too soft and their messages came too late. Women had lost agency and had lost choice. By the time the next bomb exploded, in the form of a review published in the medical journal *The Lancet*, further emphasising the HRT–breast cancer link, the collective women's health movement shrugged. *Here we go again!*

How did all this happen?

I have worked in news rooms. I understand how tough it is to explain the findings of a study, when you have just an hour to digest the press release and script the results, next to nobody to interview and another story to be written at the same time. I don't blame the journalists. But doctors let women down: from the authors of the WHI, who knew that the conclusion of the study and its accompanying press release were wrong, yet waited many years to set the record straight; to the peak bodies, who saw the study findings for what they were but were too timid to push back hard against the harmful messages, choosing instead to shout into their own tiny menopause echo-chambers. Pharmaceutical companies let women down by being so easily beaten into submission, pulling up stumps and walking away from women's health altogether.

But times, they are a-changing. Menopause seems to be having a little #MeToo moment. Finally, in the era of #TimesUp, women are standing up for themselves and each other. An unexpected side revolution has been the desire to take back the power around menopause. Let's all be a part of that movement.

Here are some interesting statistics from the UK advertising industry: women going through menopause spend 24 per cent more money on exercise and fitness than their premenopausal sisters; they spend 16 per cent more on beauty and make-up; 29 per cent more on skin care; 29 per cent more on health supplements; and 22 per cent more on travel. Does business want to ignore us? I think not. And, by the way, 76 per cent of women over 50 feel either 'very confident' or 'somewhat confident' in their own skin.

As I moved through my forties, several things happened at once that ultimately led to the writing of this book.

Being a doctor, a GP with a special interest in women's health, menopause and perimenopause are never far from my mind or my daily clinical load. But I felt increasingly ill equipped to deal with the issues my menopausal women were bringing me. Training to become a GP in the current era means I missed out on access to the information my older colleagues had about HRT. Pharma companies had slow-played the women's health market after the WHI scandal had seen the floor fall out of the HRT market. Luckily for me, I am the host of Drivetime Medical, an educational podcast for doctors that requires me to interview experts in many medical fields in Australia and around the world. Interviewing Professor Rod Baber and Dr Terri Foran (both extensively interviewed for this book) was jaw dropping in revealing both how much I didn't know, and how much is available for women suffering the symptoms of menopause. I wanted to learn more. I joined the Australian Menopause Society; I delved further into the menopause world and got hooked. There was a major story to be told here: the chasm between what was being discussed in that tiny menopause echo-chamber and what was actually happening on the ground for women was too great.

My mum, girlfriends and cousins all have their own menopause stories — the heartwarming and the horror stories. But what has struck me is the lack of formal information out there. My friends and family members, as well as my patients, are highly intelligent, well informed and proactive. So how can there be so much utter rubbish in the marketplace? Why are 'bio-identical hormones' so popular? Ditto, nutritional supplements that claim to produce a 'happy healthy you'?

Into any information void, the worst of capitalism will flow. This was rammed home to me when filming *Medicine or Myth?* for SBS — a show about home remedies and their place in medicine. I guess I already knew that menopause is a *huge* issue, but we had more submissions for menopause remedies than anything else. From what we saw, women are still suffering, in particular, from hot flushes, desperate for help and clutching at any straws for relief, either because they are terrified of taking HRT or because they can't find a doctor willing to prescribe it.

Then I hit 50. I kept being asked for advice about skin care by patients, TV viewers and readers of my blog. At the same time, I was looking for evidence-based cosmeceutical skin care for my own annoying 'combination' perimenopausal, super-sensitive, breakout prone skin. And I just couldn't find any products at all to recommend that were based on published scientific studies. It started as an itch I had to scratch and became an obsession, leading to the birth of two anti-aging skincare companies that I run with my husband, Daniel (more about these in Chapter 9, Make me look like Helen Mirren). Our customers talk to us a lot about their skin; like me, they suffer dryness and sensitivity, as well as signs of aging. Over the past few years our research has been increasingly focused on menopausal and perimenopausal skin. The new products we have developed have been specifically for women of my age, and it has made my interest in this phase of life run even deeper.

All of this is to help explain my passion for the M word. Here are a few general thoughts to bear in mind as you read.

This is all about you and your choices

I have written a book to give you access to the best information we have available today; to answer as many questions as possible; and to give you agency over your menopause journey, including the option of HRT. I'm not saying you have to take it: I have covered the lifestyle, mind-based, complementary and home remedies out there and a whole lot else, too. Many of these have some terrific evidence, and others have a good amount of anecdotal evidence. Some are shockers.

Evidence is a tricky business

The problem with anecdotal evidence (I had hot flushes, then I drank eight shots of vodka and they went away; *so, vodka cured my hot flushes*) is that there is the potential for confounding variables. For example, you drank vodka and put on a patch of HRT, too; or you drank eight shots and fell asleep and didn't feel the hot flushes because you were sauced?

There is also the potential for bias: I'd *like* to believe Mars Bars help me lose weight; I might 'feel thinner' after a Mars Bar, but objective evaluation by a third party might not validate that claim.

Scientific study requires that an event is reproducible multiple times. Good science also requires 'controlling' for 'variables'. For example, if you get five obese 75-year-olds to drink water and five thin 20-year-old netball players to drink Coke and then take their blood pressure, you might conclude that Coke is better for blood pressure than water.

Evidence also needs to exclude researcher bias as much as possible. So, if the Ponds Institute finds that Ponds has the best face cream, scientists would probably be suspicious of those findings. Research tells us that company-sponsored trials are more likely to yield positive results than independent research. Funding of research has become a fraught area — good scientific studies are very expensive, and someone needs to pay for them. Governments don't have the budgets for large studies, so it often falls to private companies to fund research. And they often won't do so unless it's financially worthwhile. That means substances such as herbs and plants often aren't well studied, because nobody can make a fortune from a herb that is widely available and not subject to patent protection. But, as

Professor Marc Cohen of RMIT Melbourne told me: 'Lack of proof of an effect is not the same as proof of lack of effect.'

Finally, to get a study published in a medical journal requires review and approval by an independent editorial board. This 'peer review' process is designed to root out puff science and the frankly fraudulent studies; the scientists need to provide proof of the studies they are writing about. It doesn't always work, but having a published study is better than one that remains unpublished (or rejected) and yet frequently discussed. This happens with some commercial products. An unpublished study of 14 people isn't 'proof'. I mention this because you will come across many 'scientifically proven' treatments for menopause in your search for help and will need to bring your sceptic's eye to the task.

So, 'evidence' is a complicated term. For many of the remedies discussed in this book, the evidence is thin and weak. That doesn't mean we *know* they don't work. We just don't know either way. As long as they're not harmful, there's often no downside to giving many complementary and alternate medicines a go. However, I will let you know if a given therapy has important side effects you need to be aware of. I have allocated these a 'Gwyneth' rating, based on the pseudoscience of a popular website that recommends the use of a vaginal steamer or carrying a jade egg inside you as a form of 'vaginal weightlifting' — something that has been criticised as having no scientific basis, no medical benefit or even being potentially harmful. My ratings range from zero Gwyneths, being reasonable, to three Gwyneths being, in my opinion, batshit crazy.

The power of placebo

Placebo is not a dirty word. Your mind can be a powerful healer. The placebo effect is based on the idea that the brain can convince the body that a non-existent treatment is actually working. There's no evidence a placebo can cure cancer or lower your cholesterol, but it can dramatically reduce your symptoms. At the end of the day, who cares what the mechanism of relief is, as long as it works? Many of my patients are completely offended by the idea that their symptoms might have responded to a placebo: in their mind that means the pain (or hot flushes) were just a figment of their imagination. Nothing could be further from the truth. The placebo effect simply shows the power of the mind–body connection. If you can get the same effect from a placebo as you can get from a drug, provided it's not more expensive or has more side effects, I can't see a problem with the placebo.

Medical and surgical menopause

In this book I have not discussed the women who have been thrown into sudden menopause, either by having both ovaries removed (for ovarian cancer, or for particular types of the BRCA gene that lead to a predisposition to cancer) or by medication (such as Tamoxifen, a medication given to women with oestrogen receptor positive breast cancer). These artificially induced pathways to menopause give far more severe symptoms and in most cases preclude HRT. I only discuss natural menopause in this book.

Other health issues

This book is specifically about menopause. So, in the interests of it not becoming too weighty a tome, I have not covered cardiovascular disease, cancer or lung disease. Not because they don't matter, but because I think those conditions are very well managed by GPs (and specialists) and I don't have much to add that will change the game for you.

Terminology

Menopause is defined as 12 months from your last menstrual period. The seven-odd years leading up to menopause is called perimenopause. This is important to understand because hormonally they are very different. I have written the chapters based on symptoms, and within each chapter I have separated out management, where it matters, into these two life phases.

Another terminology issue is HRT. In the aftermath of the WHI study, HRT had a half-hearted attempt at rebranding, calling itself MHT or 'menopause hormone therapy'. In menopause circles, we only talk about MHT these days. But outside the medical world, it's still called HRT, so that's what I've called it throughout this book, other than when it's referred to as MHT in a direct quote. They are interchangeable terms.

Find a good doctor

Finding the right doctor has never been more important. During my research, I have spoken to many women who have suffered through hot flushes and genito-urinary symptoms. Not because they didn't want HRT or even another non-hormonal medication, but because it was denied them by their doctor. This is not just GPs, but also endocrinologists managing their thinning bones and gynaecologists treating vaginal problems.

I became a GP in the era of peak hysteria around HRT after the WHI, and many of the guidelines for doctors are still tainted by the hangover of that fallout. Because of it, we were given practically no training in menopause management, so I have educated myself; you need to be highly motivated to invest the time required to get up to speed on menopause health. Prescribing medication for menopause symptoms is almost more of an art than a straightforward algorithm. I have tried to simplify it in Chapter 1, but if you are prescribed HRT by a doctor with less experience and it is just wrong for you, it can put you off the whole thing.

If, when you have finished reading this book, you don't feel your medical team is serving you well, I advise you to advocate with your doctor for access to the right treatments for you. If this doesn't work, head to the website of your country's Menopause Society and search for a member. We have not only an interest, but also experience in managing menopause. Find the right doctor for you; your wellbeing is too important to give up on.

Happy reading. Please share your own stories with me via my blog on www.drginni.com.au, Facebook, Twitter or Instagram.

CHAPTER 1

SETTING THE RECORD STRAIGHT ABOUT HRT

Oestrogen therapy is *the most effective* means of treating the symptoms of menopause. How effective? Compared with placebo, HRT has been shown in studies to reduce the frequency of hot flushes by 98 per cent and significantly reduce their severity. No other pharmacologic or alternative therapy on earth has been found to provide more relief.

And yet, many women either won't take HRT or can't, because their doctor either won't prescribe it or doesn't know how to prescribe it. What does this mean for you? If you have symptoms that are holding you back and HRT could be an option for you, keep reading. Not everybody needs, wants or can take HRT, but if you can, then you need to be armed with the facts to make the right decision about your own menopause management.

Aristotle talked about menopause, putting the age at which a woman hits that milestone as 40, but it wasn't until 1821 that a French physician coined the term 'menopause'. By the mid-nineteenth century, doctors were becoming more and more intrigued by the whole process and what caused it. In the 1930s menopause was being described as a 'deficiency disease' and doctors came up with all sorts of weird and wonderful 'cures', including 'testicular juice' and the crushed ovaries of animals.

In 1942 US pharmaceutical company Wyeth announced it was releasing an oestrogen pill of conjugated equine estrogen (CEE), called Premarin. This was seen as a saviour for newly emancipated women hoping to stay younger and healthier. Oestrogen sales doubled and tripled (other brands came to market, not just Premarin) from the mid-1960s until 1975, when studies linked the oestrogen pills with possible endometrial cancer. So researchers came up with a solution, combining the CEE with a second hormone, progestin. (Note that *progestin* is a synthetic form of your body's naturally made progesterone and is used in medications such as HRT and the Pill. *Progestogen* is an umbrella term that includes your body's own natural progesterone and synthetic progestins.) Now the treatment could claim to be both effective and safe. In 1984, a National Institutes of Health statement concluded that HRT (specifically oestrogen) was the most effective way to improve bone health in postmenopausal women. Around that time there were multiple studies seemingly showing a reduced risk of heart disease for HRT users. In the 1990s, other peak medical bodies came on board: the American Heart Association, the American College of Physicians, and the American College of Obstetricians and Gynecologists all agreed that HRT helped prevent osteoporosis and heart disease in older, postmenopausal women.

By 1992 Premarin was the top-selling drug in the US. This was backed up by a major study published in 1995 that found benefits in the cholesterol profile of HRT users. Together, these findings saw HRT assume a role as the panacea to hot flushes, night sweats and all the other menopausal symptoms we know and love.

But HRT was not just about improving hot sweats, bone health and heart health: it had become a virtual elixir of youth. Good for youthful skin, youthful lady bits and youthful bones and brains. The trend of putting almost all women on HRT was led out of the US, with pharmaceutical companies probably largely responsible. 'The physical alterations that are associated with the menopause may induce emotional changes. When a woman develops hot flushes, sweats, wrinkles on her face, she is quite concerned that she is losing her youth — that she may indeed be losing her husband,' said one company's promotional film in 1972. And *Feminine Forever*, the 1968 bestseller by New York gynaecologist Robert A. Wilson, probably hit a new low. Calling menopause 'a serious, painful and often crippling disease,' Dr Wilson, who admitted to being widely funded by the makers of HRT, insisted that HRT should be given to every woman of menopausal age. With HRT, he wrote, a woman's 'breasts and genital organs will not shrivel. She will be much more pleasant to live with and will not become dull and unattractive'.

So HRT was riding high, driven by men and their thoughts about menopause and with a fair amount of drug company money funding the movement. We shouldn't be surprised that the pendulum would swing back and swing hard. The whole business unravelled through a series of events that have left women back at square one, with far less access to options for menopausal symptoms.

Why did it all go wrong?

It was in 2002 that everything changed.

This was when the hormone replacement therapy subgroup (the other subgroups were diet modification, and calcium and vitamin D supplements) of the enormous US-based Women's Health Initiative (WHI) Study was abruptly stopped early, after only 5.6 years, with enormous media attention. The researchers had apparently found an increase in breast cancer and heart disease with combination HRT (oestrogen plus progestogen). The way the study and these findings were reported changed everything.

The WHI was, by any standards, a massive study. Overall, 161,000 women between the ages of 50 and 79 years participated (doctors *love* a big study). It was also a randomised, prospective (so moving forwards rather than looking backwards) placebo-controlled trial — doctors absolutely *love* this over the less reliable, retrospective analysis (that looks back once an outcome is known, to determine what factors might have led to it).

Dr Tim Hillard is the Trustee and Past Chair of the British Menopause Society. Dr Hillard said that, until WHI, doctors all around the world had believed HRT was a low-risk and very positive intervention for women. The Nurses' Health Study and the 2002 Cache County Study had shown that

HRT might help prevent not just heart disease and osteoporosis, but dementia as well. But these were side benefits: the purpose of HRT was the treatment of menopause symptoms, especially hot flushes and vaginal and bladder symptoms.

The WHI was designed to find out whether older women who started on HRT after menopause (i.e., not for its intended purpose of managing menopausal symptoms) would enjoy the same heart-health benefits as younger women who started taking it during peak menopause symptoms. So, the WHI study intentionally didn't include many recently menopausal women. Well, we already knew about the benefits to them, didn't we? The average age of the women starting on HRT in the WHI was 63. But 25 per cent of them were over 70 when they started their HRT. And, this is important: the women on HRT in this trial were older than the women on placebo, with 66.6 per cent of the women in the HRT group being between 60 and 79 years. That is almost unheard of in clinical practice, but they were trying to determine whether the cardiovascular benefits of HRT meant you're 'never too old' to start. The researchers didn't measure quality of life or reduction in flushes for the women in the study, because the HRT was being looked at as a cardiovascular disease preventer only.

The women were chosen at random to take either Prempro (0.625mg CEE and 2.5mg medroxyprogesterone acetate, or CEE alone if they'd had a previous hysterectomy) or placebo. They were going to be followed up for 15 years but instead the WHI was terminated early, in July 2002, because of some negative results for the women on HRT.

It's also worth pointing out that Prempro is a form of HRT that I would basically *never* prescribe today. There are now *many* types of HRT and these days, with access to transdermal oestrogen and micronised progesterone, both of which have much lower side effects, few women would be on these older formulations.

What were the WHI results?

No one can reasonably argue that the trial should have been continued at the time, because to do so would have been reckless. But, the conclusions were incorrect and reflected in large part the inherent skew in the trial.

More heart attacks

There was a reported 29 per cent increase in heart attacks in the HRT group compared with the placebo group. This means that for every 10,000 person-years (10,000 women taking it for one year) there would be 37 women who had a heart attack while on HRT, compared to 30 women having heart attacks on placebo. That means seven more women out of 10,000 in a year.

Don't get me wrong: that's bad if you are one of the seven. But, not only is that a tiny increase, don't forget that the HRT group was older than the placebo group, so you would expect a higher risk. And, furthermore, you need to remember this was in women who started a form of HRT most doctors no longer use, often at an age when most women would be well and truly off HRT already.

In 2008 the data from WHI was put through the ringer once again to adjust for some of these differences, and the study data actually showed that the younger women in the study (the women who started HRT around the time of menopause) had a *reduced* heart disease risk.

More strokes

The headline reported a 41 per cent increase in strokes in the women taking HRT, compared to the women on placebo. There were in fact 29 cases of stroke in women on HRT versus 21 in women on placebo per 10,000 person-years. That meant eight more women in 10,000. Plus the caveats I mentioned above.

But even this headline was a distortion of the study findings. There were, as reported, more cardiovascular events in the women receiving HRT *in the first two years after starting their HRT*. But this literally flipped around after two years, when the women on HRT actually had *fewer* 'adverse cardiovascular end points' (heart attacks, strokes and blood clots in the legs and lungs) than the women taking placebo. This meant that overall, there were no differences in cardiovascular end points between the two groups by the end of the study.

More breast cancer

This was the Biggie. The one that caught the media attention. The study found a 26 per cent increase in the risk of breast cancer among women on HRT compared to placebo. That translated to 38 women per 10,000 per year in the women on HRT, compared to 30 women per 10,000 in the women on placebo.

Now remember that this is an increased risk of breast cancer for women who started taking HRT long after menopause. When the data was re-examined to look at women who started HRT *during* menopause, it actually showed *no* increased risk in breast cancer.

So, apart from this headline error, let me put the stated risk into perspective. For this older group of women, the risk of breast cancer from using HRT is slightly higher than the risk (found by the same study) of drinking one glass of wine a night, but *less* than the risk of drinking two glasses of wine a night. The risk of breast cancer from taking HRT in these older women was similar to the risk reported with obesity and low physical activity. I find it ironic that so many of my patients are terrified of taking HRT for their hot flushes but continue to enjoy wine o'clock and might be well over their healthy weight range. I am certainly not judging, because I *love* my wine and my weight is a constant harrowing battle for me, but nobody is terrified of that second glass of wine the way they are of HRT.

The other thing to keep in perspective is cancer risk altogether. Between 35–40 per cent of women in developed countries die of cardio-vascular disease. And 20–25 per cent of women die of cancer (any cancer). 'We need to be aware of cancer, not to fear it,' says Professor Anne Gompel, Head of Gynaecological Endocrinology at Université Paris Descartes. 'It is important to understand that the increase in cancer incidence is related at least partially to increasing life expectancy — the older a woman becomes, the more time there is for a cancer to develop. Increasing use of cancer screening also means that more cancers are being picked up than in previous years.'

Some positive effects

The study also reported a 37 per cent decrease in the risk of bowel or colorectal cancer for women on HRT. Ten women per 10,000 per year developed colorectal cancer on HRT, versus 16 women per 10,000 per year taking placebo. There was also a 34 per cent decrease in the risk of hip fracture, a key measure of osteoporosis. The study saw 10 hip fractures in women on HRT per 10,000 per year versus 15 in the placebo group.

What was wrong with the WHI findings?

The authors concluded: 'The risk–benefit profile found in this trial is not consistent with the requirements for a viable intervention for primary prevention of chronic diseases, and the results indicate that this regimen should not be initiated or continued for primary prevention of coronary heart disease.'

The research was good; the headlines around it were not. Remember, this was a study of older women who often didn't have symptoms of menopause, looking for cardiovascular protection. Yet, the results were reported as if it were a standard HRT regimen with results that could be applied to women in their forties and fifties. Tying the results found in older women to younger women twisted the entire logic of the study. Younger women, the group who actually *needed* HRT the most, were thrown under the bus.

There were many, albeit faint, voices at the time that were critical of the study's conclusion and the way it emphasised some of the more sensationalist results and buried the more benign data. Nobody took much notice, until *finally* we heard from someone who knew firsthand what had happened inside the WHI walls. Professor Robert D. Langer was one of the authors of the original study. In 2017 he broke his silence. Unlike many of his fellow authors, who had over the years blamed the media reporting of the data for the spread of misinformation, Professor Langer described in the prestigious journal *Climacteric* what had really happened.

He revealed that in June 2002, he and other WHI investigators had gathered for one of their regular editorial meetings in Chicago. They were told that the combination HRT arm of the trial was being shut down early. Langer says the decision was 'based on a finding of likely futility', meaning that the combination HRT didn't actually have the benefits they were expecting. There was no mention of any harm from HRT at that stage.

Can you imagine the horror of this group of researchers when they discovered a secretly written initial results paper and a press release with completely different information? Information that was not actually reflective of the study results? In fact, the initial paper and press release had been written by a small subgroup of study authors, who declared an increase in breast cancer as the reason they were terminating the trial. Plus, they said, there was also an increase in heart attacks. According to Professor Langer, the article, with all its drama and negative results and conclusion, was kept secret from the vast majority of scientists in whose names it was submitted, until after it was accepted by the highly prestigious *Journal of the American Medical Association* (*JAMA*).

The researchers gathered at that Chicago meeting quickly tried to draft changes to the article. These were couriered to *JAMA*, but it was too late: the journal had been printed with the original piece. And journalists were off to the races with this incredible story that HRT causes breast cancer and heart disease. The rest of the authors thought the paper's conclusions misrepresented the scientific findings and made exaggerated, inflammatory claims, but they felt there was nothing they could do.

What happened after WHI?

Headlines screamed about the deadly breast-cancer-causing consequences of HRT. The result was widespread panic. Women threw their HRT patches and tablets in the bin; many felt sick to discover that what had been prescribed by their doctor to keep them healthy was supposedly 'deadly'. Doctors refused to prescribe HRT, telling women to live with their hot flushes. And the belief that HRT is deadly, stuck. Even discussing The M Word was just not done anymore. It became a taboo.

As Dr Tim Hillard pointed out to me, this all happened in the era before social media, so broadcast media and newspapers were the only messages that went out to the public. 'I'd be interested to know what would happen if the study was released now,' he told me. I don't know. I think in our Facebook era, beliefs that Big Pharma companies are in cahoots to make people sick are even more pervasive than they ever were.

Anyway, the use of HRT to treat menopausal symptoms plummeted by as much as 80 per cent. A study published in 2013 estimated that 91,610 women died prematurely between 2002 and 2012 in the US as a result of declining to take HRT to relieve symptoms of menopause. The extra deaths came primarily from increased cardiovascular disease, but also non-breast cancer (for example, colorectal cancer).

Governments fail

After the events of 2002, both the US and UK governments immediately issued new guidelines, stating that the only reason women and their doctors should consider HRT would be for treatment of 'moderate to severe' symptoms of menopause, such as moderate to severe hot flushes or significant risk of osteoporosis fracture. And then HRT should be used at the lowest possible dose and for the shortest amount of time.

In January 2003, they went further. The US Food and Drug Administration (FDA) demanded that labels be placed on HRT packages. The labels were to carry a 'black box' warning about the increased risk of heart disease, heart attack, stroke and breast cancer. That sounds serious. If my government put out a warning that a drug will harm me, I'd probably toughen up and soldier on without it. Especially since hot flushes were seen as a 'lifestyle issue'. The warnings are still in place today on HRT in all forms, including vaginal oestrogen creams and pessaries, which are used only for vaginal symptoms of menopause with no evidence that they have any effect on breast cancer risk or ever have had.

The legal system fails

Drug companies started getting sued after WHI was shut down early. The money was big and the lawsuits were successful. The juries in these trials were asked to adjudicate on some pretty technical issues. Is it any surprise that the journal article headlines held sway?

Wyeth faced thousands of lawsuits over its HRT formulations. Famously, in 2007, US$3 million was awarded to the husband of a woman who died of breast cancer after taking Prempro, which Wyeth manufactured and marketed. A bunch of trials followed and Wyeth was sued for around US$20 million altogether. Wyeth ended up being sold to Pfizer in 2009, and they inherited even more lawsuits. Pfizer is rumoured to have agreed to pay $US330 million as a lump sum to resolve the claims. HRT was now a giant pain in the butt. The investment in research and development for menopause effectively dried up. Investment into women's health generally was just largely ignored.

Journalists fail

Respected women's health journalist and activist Barbara Seaman is well known for her bestselling 2003 book, *The Greatest Experiment Ever Performed on Women: Exploding the Estrogen Myth*. In the book, she looked at the HRT–cancer link reported in the initial WHI headlines and concluded that drug companies such as Wyeth, and Schering in Germany, were guilty of putting profits above the wellbeing of women. She fed into the belief that Big Pharma conspires to hide the adverse effects of their products, and cares only about money.

Doctors fail

Professor Rodney Baber is past president of the International Menopause Society (IMS), Editor-in-Chief of *Climacteric* journal and lead author of the IMS recommendations on HRT. I have interviewed him countless times about menopause and HRT for various podcasts and publications. When I decided to write this book, he was the first person I turned to.

Professor Baber says the tragedy surrounding the WHI study was both for the women who became terrified of the therapy that in many cases was helping them, and for the generation of GPs, endocrinologists and even gynaecologists left too scared to prescribe HRT, and then ultimately without the knowledge, confidence and experience to do so. As a result, their patients now have fewer choices in managing their menopause symptoms as the big treatment has been taken off the table.

To this day, women coming into my practice seem to regard needing treatment for their hot flushes as a sign of weakness. If I suggest that one option is to give HRT a go ('You're not getting married to it, you can just give it a shot and see how you go . . .'), they often keep it a secret. They don't tell their sisters and friends for fear of being castigated as weak, or as stooges for Big Pharma, taking dangerous drugs that will give them breast cancer and kill them. Many are not even prepared to consider it. If you are suffering from symptoms of menopause, you should feel free to ask for HRT from your doctor. And you shouldn't feel guilty about taking it or feel you need to hide it from your friends and family.

One of my girlfriends is my age. She was struggling with hot flushes and insomnia, and her libido had fallen off a cliff. She'd also put on about 6kg in a year — she couldn't exercise due to the flushes. Every time I saw her she had a fan in one hand and would constantly apologise as she wiped her wet brow and chin with a hanky. I asked her what she was doing about it. It turns out she'd gone to discuss her symptoms with her GP six months earlier. Her GP is in her forties and evidently a fantastic family doctor. So, when the GP told her the answer was to 'lose weight', my friend took that on board. She gave it her best shot. She lost a kilo. The flushes got worse. She wasn't getting more than two consecutive hours of sleep at night, so she went back to the GP and asked her directly for HRT. Her GP warned her off it. 'There's the risk of breast cancer and heart disease. If you want that you'll need to see a specialist — I'm not prescribing it.'

I restrained myself from badmouthing her GP. Instead, I offered the names of gynaecologists who might be able to give her 'some options'. I saw her the other day: she was started on HRT by one of the gurus I interviewed for this book. Not only is she not having even one hot flush, but she's also lost the weight and feels like a different person. I know her GP is fantastic: she has given outstanding care to my friend's children, she never prescribes antibiotics unnecessarily and has managed my friend's husband's heart-disease risks according to the very best guidelines. And she is lovely and my friend trusts her implicitly. You can't put a price on that. Menopause is just a black hole for her, as for so many doctors. Other women who are faced with unbearable hot flushes and a doctor who won't countenance prescribing HRT are driven to the fringe sector of doctors who prescribe bio-identical hormones (which are just another form of HRT, even though doctors who prescribe and sell them say they're not). Bio-identical hormones are made by a compounding pharmacist, rather than a drug company, which means nobody's checking them, whereas pharmaceutical companies have government regulators constantly and thoroughly checking.

Dr Tim Hillard told me that in the UK there is an entire generation of doctors trained in the 2000s who have had very little exposure to prescribing HRT. It's not that all doctors are labouring under the misconception that HRT is dangerous, but many don't know what therapy to prescribe, at what dose or how to tailor it to the patient's needs. If a patient comes back with a HRT-related problem, such as sore breasts, weight gain, low mood or vaginal bleeding, doctors who don't have the experience to manage these problems might just abandon ship rather than try to adjust the regimen.

This is partly because of the lack of education in HRT. Drug company-sponsored education for doctors around menopause is practically non-existent these days. There are few educational activities. Most medical schools completely ignore menopause; in fact, a US survey found that only one in five training programs for obstetricians and gynaecologists provided any kind of menopause training whatsoever. Unless your doctor becomes a member of your country or region's Menopause Society (I'm a member of the Australian Menopause Society, AMS), they're likely to be a bit thin on knowledge.

There's another problem. Doctors are incredibly conservative by nature and we are terrified of being sued. The practice of defensive medicine deserves a book of its own, but GPs and even gynaecologists worry that, even though the initial reporting of the WHI was dead wrong, a jury of peers without training in critical scientific reasoning would convict the doctor of negligence if a woman on HRT developed breast cancer. It happens often, and the payouts are in the millions of dollars. It feels safer not to even go there. I get it: I would hate to be sued. And I'd hate to be unfairly convicted based on bad science and misinformation tainting a jury's view of my clinical practice. I'd hate to have my practice wiped out because of it.

But all of that doesn't change the fact that women are the biggest losers here. This has all led to a complete failure in managing menopause and the menopause consultation. A Yale University review of insurance claims from more than 500,000 women at various stages of menopause found that 60 per cent with troubling symptoms actually do seek help from a doctor. But only a quarter get treatment! Prescribing HRT can be more of an art than managing, say, high blood pressure, for which we have really simple algorithms, so it's easy to see why the HRT many women end up on is not quite right and can cause more issues than it fixes.

The Menopause Societies fail

After a huge amount of behind-the-scenes collaboration, in 2013, a ridiculous 11 years after the WHI shutdown, the International Menopause Society released its Global Consensus Statement on Menopausal Hormone Therapy. It was released in conjunction with the North American Menopause Society (NAMS), the Endocrine Society, the European Menopause and Andropause Society, the Asia Pacific Menopause Federation, the International Osteoporosis Foundation and the Federation of Latin American Menopause Societies. Collectively, they said:

'MHT . . . is the most effective treatment for vasomotor symptoms [hot flushes] associated with menopause at any age, but benefits are more likely to outweigh risks if initiated for symptomatic women before the age of 60 years or within 10 years after menopause.'

To me, the language was still too guarded. The statement got no publicity whatsoever; it wasn't even really heard by most doctors. It didn't change the black box warnings on all forms of HRT. And maybe that's why 2013 certainly didn't see a turnaround in the acceptance of HRT by women and their doctors.

Gynaecologist Dr Nicholas Panay is the General Secretary of the International Menopause Society, the President of The Royal Society of Medicine (O&G Division) and Director of the International Centre for Hormone Health in London. He agrees that Menopause Societies need to be doing more. 'We need changes in health policy, we need public meetings, celebrity engagement, we need more advocacy groups,' he said.

More bad news

Just as more of my patients were coming around to the idea of accepting help for their menopausal symptoms, another bombshell dropped. In September

2019 the prestigious medical journal *The Lancet* published a review article teasing out the relationship between HRT and breast cancer. The review looked at women diagnosed with breast cancer between January 1992 and January 2018, and comprised data from 58 studies of 108,647 postmenopausal women. In this study, 51 per cent of the women who developed breast cancer had used HRT, and 85 per cent of them were overweight or obese.

The report confirmed the small increase in the risk of breast cancer from taking HRT. Once again, that risk was highest with combination oestrogen and progestogen HRT, but for the first time the authors found a slight increased risk from oestrogen-only HRT. This is interesting, but hasn't changed recommendations of Menopause Societies. It is a retrospective (less scientifically robust) analysis of HRT in doses and regimens that are rarely used these days.

I received an email from the Australian Menopause Society on the same day the study came out. The International, British and North American Menopause Societies were equally proactive. This time, they were on the front foot in trying to avert any potential panic.

Here are the takeaway points from this study:

- The study confirmed the small increased risk of breast cancer from HRT use.
- The increased risk of breast cancer needs to be seen in the context of the significant improvement in quality of life for women who suffer the symptoms of menopause, as well as the decrease in heart disease for women who start using HRT around the time of menopause, and the better bone health from HRT.
- Once again, the HRT regimens used in the women who developed breast cancer in this study were different from those currently recommended.
- Once again, in this study alcohol and obesity conferred a higher risk of breast cancer than HRT.

To a certain extent, so much damage to HRT's reputation had been done back in 2002 that this article just went into the 'here we go again' file.

It was reported, but didn't make the same front-page news as the 2002 study. Anecdotally, there hasn't been the same panicked response and none of my patients appear to have binned their HRT yet.

What about the future?

Change is coming, with social movements empowering women to demand access to a great menopause. Led by celebrities such as Kim Cattrall, Emma Thompson, Gillian Anderson, Angelina Jolie, Yasmin Le Bon, Jean Kittson and Davina McCall, women are starting to come out as menopausal (as if we didn't know a woman approaching 60 might have gone through a bit of a change). With the #TimesUp and #MeToo movements, investment by companies in women's health might be starting to slowly crank up again. As one pharmaceutical exec put it: 'The voice of the patient is getting louder. Women want better treatments in a field that has been largely ignored.' KaNDy Therapeutics, a UK-based bio-tech company, has announced promising results for a new once-daily pill known as NT-814, in women with debilitating menopausal symptoms. Early trial results found 84 per cent reduction in the number of hot flushes from baseline (with 37 per cent reduction for placebo) in two weeks. Plus less severe hot flushes and fewer night-time wake-ups.

Women of menopausal age are a powerful consumer group. What they want matters. They're not going to sit around sweating, or throw away their sex lives, without demanding access to treatment. They're growing in confidence, too. I've also noticed that, as women make up a larger percentage of GPs and gynaecologists, and as more women doctors reach an age (like me!) when this is all incredibly relevant, and as peak bodies try to change opinion about HRT, finally the message is getting through. We're seeing a resurgence of GPs, and even gynaecologists, prepared to prescribe HRT for their patients and doing it really well. We just need to hurry up and grow our numbers, because until we do, women are turning to whoever they can for answers — online bloggers and influencers, Dr Google and bio-identical hormone peddlars — and they're not the best candidates.

WHI revisited — is opinion slowly turning?

Since it was published, there has been ever-increasing criticism of the way the data in the WHI was put together into a published paper. In fact, as Langer and countless organisations have pointed out, when you reanalyse the data, as many researchers have now done, the study showed a small increase in the risk of breast cancer and no increase in heart disease risk in women using HRT.

In 2017 the data from the WHI trial was re-examined by different researchers and published in *JAMA*. The conclusion? Let me quote:

'Among postmenopausal women, hormone therapy with conjugated equine estrogens (CEE) plus medroxyprogesterone acetate (MPA) for a median of 5.6 years or with CEE alone for a median of 7.2 years was not associated with risk of all-cause, cardiovascular or cancer mortality during a cumulative follow-up of 18 years.'

I'll go even further. More late analysis of WHI data shows that if you look only at women between the ages of 50 and 59, when most women use it and need it, there are clear benefits of HRT. These women had *fewer* cancers, fractures and deaths from any cause compared to the women taking placebo.

There are exceptions and, as we drill down into the data, there are particular women who might have a bit more to worry about. A presentation to the European Menopause Society in 2019 by Professor Anne Gompel was webcast to all members of Menopause Societies around the world, including mine — the Australian Menopause Society. She presented a data-rich analysis of the link between HRT and breast cancer, and pointed out that in some women with some early breast cancers, the HRT might promote these cancers.

She advised women to know their personal breast-cancer risk. All of these increase your risk of breast cancer fourfold or more:

- Known BRCA mutation
- High family history of breast cancer (*more than one* first-degree relative: mother, sister, daughter)
- A previous biopsy of a lump that showed a non-cancerous problem such as ductal carcinoma in situ (DCIS) or 'atypical hyperplasia'

- Previous radiotherapy to the chest, especially as a child
- Very high breast density on 3D mammogram (classified as Birad d).

None of these factors are common. And it's not that these women should *not* take HRT, but that their risk of breast cancer is higher and they should make a choice armed with that information.

Have I convinced you? For most women HRT is safe and effective. I'm not saying you *have* to take it; far from it. But you should have a choice.

What do I need to know about HRT?

Because there is an, albeit smaller than initially reported, increased risk of blood clots and breast cancer for some older women on some types of HRT, we don't put it in the water for everyone — it is used as a treatment for specific menopause-related problems. To clarify that risk, for breast cancer, the risk is around nine additional breast cancer cases for every 10,000 person-years of HRT. That is a risk slightly greater than drinking a glass of wine daily, but less than two glasses of wine. It's around the same risk as obesity and low physical activity. And for a form of HRT we almost never use anymore; modern forms have a lower risk. Compared with placebo, HRT seems to be linked to an extra six strokes per 10,000 women.

Unlike treating cholesterol, asthma or high blood pressure, there is a bit of an art to prescribing HRT. Professor Bronwyn Stuckey is a Perth-based endocrinologist; she describes choosing HRT as 'like trying on a dress'. Everyone has different priorities and in an ideal world the doctor and patient would collaborate around your priorities, your health history and risk factors as well as your preferences. So, whether you want to take HRT for your menopause symptoms or for your bone health, my intention is to help you make a choice about what kind of HRT is right for you.

Combination or oestrogen-only HRT?

It is the oestrogen in hormone therapy that does the heavy lifting in terms of getting rid of hot flushes, other menopause-related symptoms and bone loss. However, if you have a uterus (i.e., you haven't had a hysterectomy) and you take oestrogen alone without its hormone sister, progesterone, you increase the risk of a condition called endometrial hyperplasia (overgrowth of the lining of the uterus) and endometrial cancer.

Therefore, *all* women with a uterus must take a progestogen along with their oestrogens to protect their endometrium. This is called combination HRT.

But if you have had a hysterectomy, your need for progesterone disappears and you can take oestrogen-only HRT. Oestrogen-only HRT has never been linked to heart disease or clots in any study. And breast cancer risk was lower in the WHI. The 2019 *Lancet* article, finding the slightly higher breast cancer risk for women on oestrogen-only HRT, is at this stage an outlier and guidelines have not been changed.

Cyclical or continuous HRT?

Combined HRT comes in two forms. You can take 'cyclical' (also called 'sequential') HRT, in which the oestrogen is given daily and the progestogen is given 10–14 days of the month. With cyclical HRT you will have a withdrawal bleed (which is similar to, but not technically, a menstrual period).

The alternative is 'continuous' HRT, in which both oestrogen and progestogen are given daily. Continuous HRT should not give you a bleed.

We use cyclical HRT for women who are perimenopausal, still having periods, but still need some help to control hot flushes. Cyclical HRT is also used if it's less than a year since your last period, because you can get a bit of breakthrough bleeding if we start continuous HRT too early. That breakthrough bleeding can be really annoying, if nothing else. While HRT will relieve the hot flushes, it's not as high a hormone dose as the pill and can't promise to stop you ovulating, so if you are perimenopausal and sexually active, you will need to use other contraception.

Different doses?

Dr Terri Foran is a lecturer with the School of Women's and Children's Health at the University of New South Wales and is the Director of Master Women's Health Medicine. 'In the past there was a lot of pressure to put women on the lowest dose [of HRT] possible for the least possible time,' she told me. These days, in light of the re-crunched WHI study data, we start at a medium oestrogen dose and titrate down if we have to. It's because medium doses are statistically more likely to settle the hot flushes and you might as well take a dose that works.

Different HRT delivery systems?

HRT comes in a few forms. You can get a combo pack of HRT pills or patches containing both oestrogen and progestogen. Or you can separate the two hormones out. If you're separating them (and this is what I prefer in 90 per cent of cases, as I will explain below), you can get your oestrogens in the form of tablets, skin patches, gels and sprays. You can also get oestrogen in vaginal creams, pessaries or tablets that are better for vaginal dryness but won't be enough to curb hot flushes.

All progestogens can be taken orally in a tablet. Some types can also be absorbed through the skin so can be added to an oestrogen patch. In some forms it can be placed directly into the vagina as well. It can also be packed into an IUD and delivered directly to the uterus. This is a super common way of delivering progesterone to where it is needed most, especially for perimenopausal women, because it covers your progesterone needs and gives you awesome contraception at the same time. It is the method I chose for myself and I'll talk more about this throughout the book.

I tend not to prescribe oestrogen tablets first, even though they are the cheapest way to get your HRT. Patches or gels seem to work better for women who have issues with their moods, triglycerides (one of the measures of cholesterol) and for women at higher risk of developing blood clots; for example, women who are overweight or smokers.

ORAL HRT	TRANSDERMAL HRT (PATCHES, CREAMS, GELS AND SPRAYS)
Daily	Once or twice a week; daily spray
Can cause nausea	Nausea is rare
No skin reaction	Some women get rashes from the glue that holds the patches to the skin
Seems to have a higher risk of weight gain, bloating, breast tenderness	Less of all of that
Increased clotting risk (except Tibolone)	No higher clotting risk

What are oestrogens in HRT?

(Firstly, a note about confusing spellings! Oestrogen/oestradiol is the UK and Australian–English spelling; estrogen/estradiol is the US spelling. And, because Americans have led much of the research, the acronyms have their E spellings.)

Broadly speaking, there are three types of oestrogen: conjugated equine estrogens (CEE), ethinyl estradiol (EE), and micronised 17beta estradiol (E2). Most doctors veer towards E2 as our oestrogen of choice in HRT. While all three forms are steroid hormones, CEE and E2 are classified as natural oestrogens and EE as a synthetic oestrogen. But in reality only E2 is *truly* a natural oestrogen. (Both CEE and EE have components that are not found in women but do have oestrogen-like activity.) The E2 used in menopause formulations is made from a compound called diosgenin, which is found naturally in yams and soy beans. EE is made from plant steroids and is biochemically very similar to E2, only much stronger.

A systematic review of 32 randomised trials confirmed that CEE and E2 had both significant and also comparable effects on the treatment of menopausal hot flushes. But studies show that women using oestradiol generally have a lower risk of blood clots and heart attacks than women using CEE. Both EE and CEE increase triglyceride levels, while E2 (either orally or transdermal) does not.

What are progestogens in HRT?

A popular delivery method is the progestin-containing IUD, especially for perimenopausal women who are still having periods. This contains one of the older progestins — levonorgestrel — which acts in the uterus alone to prevent the effects of oestrogen on the endometrium. In around 5 per cent of women, systemic absorption leads to headaches, acne, breast tenderness or depression. In studies, the incidence of these effects usually peaked at three months after insertion and then declined.

When it comes to progestins, the older types (like the medroxy-progesterone acetate, MPA, used in the WHI trial) seem to activate the glucocorticoid receptors in the body along with the progesterone receptors.

This could account for some of the side effects, such as mood swings and swelling of feet, and occasionally the hands, too.

I tend to prescribe the newer progesterones, such as micronised or 'body identical' progesterone or dydrogesterone (Duphaston). There are a few reasons for this. Firstly, observational studies from France and Finland show that these forms of progesterone absolutely don't cause any increase in breast cancer risk as compared to the conclusions from studies, including the WHI, around medroxyprogesterone acetate (MPA).

Secondly, in the case of micronised progesterone, there is some flexibility in the way it can be used. You can take it orally, like any other tablet. One big advantage of this is that, if you take it at night, it improves your sleep quality. All progesterone does this, as it is a bit of a sedative, but the micronised progesterone seems to do it a little better.

You can also insert the tablet directly into the vagina, like a pessary. Some of my patients tell me it gives a bit of a discharge; however, because it is only needed three times a week when taken this way, it works out at less than half the price of taking it nightly. On cost alone, this is a very popular way of using micronised progesterone, although I still get many perplexed calls from pharmacists asking whether I wrote that instruction by accident! To reassure, I point them to the Australian Menopause Society and International Menopause Society webpages addressing this. Lastly, micronised progesterone doesn't activate the glucocorticoid receptors in the body so has less side effects.

For most women who experience problems from their HRT, such as moodiness, bloating, breast tenderness or foot swelling, the issues are related to the progestogen they're taking. I often find that changing their progesterone sorts out these symptoms (in almost every case this means either switching to a micronised progesterone or using a progesterone-containing IUD).

What are selective oestrogen receptor modulators (SERMs)?

These drugs literally sit on some oestrogen receptors and not others. None activate receptors in the endometrium, so don't need to be paired with progesterones. Some, like Tamoxifen, are used to *block* oestrogen receptors in the breast. So they are used to treat, and in some cases prevent, breast cancer. They usually make hot flushes, aches and pains, and vaginal symptoms worse, so have *no role* outside prevention and management of breast cancer. Raloxifene works on oestrogen receptors in bones so does great stuff for women with osteoporosis and can reduce the risk of breast cancer by 70 per cent. But, like Tamoxifen, it can make menopause symptoms worse. Bazedoxifene is a third-generation SERM and is combined with oestrogen (CEE) at a moderate dose. It helps prevent osteoporosis and can really help with menopause symptoms. Although for hot flushes, this combo is less effective than standard HRT in studies.

Putting all of this together, I have drawn a table (shown opposite) to help you choose the right HRT, based on your individual concerns and priorities.

Is there anyone who can't take HRT?

There are women who simply cannot take HRT, ever. This is you, if:

- You (*not* your mum or your sister) have a previous history of oestrogen receptor positive breast cancer
- You have coronary heart disease
- You have had a previous blood clot in your lung, leg or pelvis, or a stroke or a clotting problem that makes you prone to developing blood clots
- You have uncontrolled high blood pressure
- You currently have liver disease (chat to your GP if you're not sure; a couple of abnormal liver tests due to excess weight is okay).

What about side effects of HRT?

It's not uncommon for a patient to tell me she's tried HRT but it 'didn't work for me'. Didn't work? Are you sure? What she actually means is that she developed intolerable side effects from the HRT and, when she went

SITUATION	HRT
Perimenopause	Low-dose contraception OR cyclical HRT (if you have another form of contraception) OR continuous oestrogen HRT with progesterone-containing IUD
Worried about weight gain	Transdermal HRT
Breast pain or enlargement	Transdermal HRT, or lower the HRT dose, or switch to a SERM/oestrogen combo such as Tibolone (page 60)
Low libido	Try Tibolone, but in my experience it is better in theory than practice. Testosterone cream is great for this
Any heart disease/diabetes or high cholesterol or high risk of these conditions	Transdermal HRT
Migraines	Continuous therapy (not cyclical) and transdermal HRT are better than tablets
Mood problems (or a history of mood problems)	Micronised progesterone only. But either patches or oral oestrogen is OK
You don't want anyone to see a patch on your body, skin is irritated by glue of the patches or you just don't like patches	Oral HRT or one of the oestrogen gel or spray formulations
Forgetful about taking pills, etc	Combination oestrogen and progesterone patch that you change twice weekly

back to the GP, was just told to stop the therapy altogether. That results in women dealing with mood swings, hot flushes and the rest when just a few tweaks to the dose, formulation or delivery method could have fixed things up pretty quickly.

The table on the following page lists the common side effects and how to combat them, so that you don't end up 'failing' on HRT.

SIDE EFFECTS	REMEDY
Breakthrough bleeding	Are you remembering to take your HRT every day? Compliance is essential! If it's less than 12 months from your last period and you're on a continuous HRT regimen, this is expected. I would switch you to a cyclical regimen until you're a year from your last period. If it's more than 12 months from your last period and you're on a continuous HRT regimen, you need to see a gynaecologist to rule out any sinister cause. Often this is nothing sinister and is just a matter of tweaking the dosage of the oestrogen, progesterone or both.
Nausea	Less common on transdermal oestrogen (such as patches) and with lower doses of oestrogen.
Bloating	Switching to micronised progesterone (if you're currently taking another form) seems to help. Check in with your doctor, especially if you have had a change of bowel habits and/or blood in your stools.
Breast tenderness	This is common on HRT. If you're on conjugated equine oestrogen, switch to oestradiol or transdermal oestrogen. Both give less breast tenderness. Or switch to an oestrogen/bazedoxifene combo, which seems to cause less breast tenderness. I get fewer reports of breast tenderness when I prescribe the micronised progesterone as a vaginal tablet three times a week, rather than orally every night. I have no studies to back this up, but other studies have found that reducing progesterone dose over the month (for example, using cyclical HRT) has been related to fewer complaints of breast pain than continuous progesterone. But reducing the progesterone dose over the month will give you your periods back — so that might be a 'no thanks'!
Migraines	Less common with transdermal oestrogen (e.g., patches). Studies show higher doses of oestrogen cause less migraines than lower doses.
Mood swings	Switch your progesterone to dydrogesterone or micronised progesterone, which have less effect on mood.

How long can I stay on HRT?

After the WHI study, the advice was to take 'the lowest dose possible for the shortest time possible'. That is now completely dismissed. Most menopause specialists (and every expert I spoke to, without exception) say you can use HRT indefinitely, being cognisant of the small risks associated with using it when you're older. Because the benefits outweigh the risks. Caveats: start HRT within 10 years of the start of your menopause and get a regular review from your doctor (I do it yearly).

The experts I spoke to mostly agreed that the length of time you stay on HRT depends on what you're trying to achieve. *All* the experts (even those who still take the WHI at face value without looking at the new interpretation of the data) agree that using HRT for three years *only* will not in any way increase your risk of breast cancer. Use it to treat symptoms of menopause such as hot flushes and anxiety, when those symptoms are at their worst, within the first 10 years of menopause. Some women choose to stop then, because they fear any hint of cancer risk and that is more important to them than symptom relief. I understand that and am happy to support this choice.

But I and most menopause experts explain to them that if your main concern is controlling the symptoms of menopause (such as hot flushes, dry vagina, low libido or mood swings) you can choose to use HRT for as long as your symptoms last. For some women, this is forever. As I have explained, the risk is low. But many women don't want to be on a medication they don't need. And they are happy to take it, but would prefer not to if they don't have to.

A problem with this use-it-until-you-don't-need-it-anymore strategy is that you won't have symptoms while you're on HRT. So the only way to know whether the flushes are still lurking is to try coming off it.

There's no consensus here, but at a patient's annual check-up, around four to five years after starting HRT, I often suggest she switches to a lower dose of oestrogen and checks out what happens. Coming off HRT will see your body reset to where it would have been if you'd never started it. Hot flushes, vaginal symptoms, mood symptoms and bone strength will reset. You might then choose to resume HRT.

How do I come off HRT?

The official answer is that we have no consensus on how to stop HRT. Should you go cold turkey or slowly wean off it? Studies tell us that hot flushes come back for 50 per cent of women when they stop HRT, regardless of whether they come off it suddenly or slowly. We're not sure whether this is because, without HRT on board, you're back where you would have been if you hadn't been taking the HRT for this time. Or whether the withdrawal of oestrogen causes the flushes and, had you never been on HRT, the whole flushing thing would have disappeared years ago.

Now the real answer: no expert would ever suggest going cold turkey off HRT. I chatted about this with Dr Terri Foran and her opinion was clear: she would always wean you off slowly. She recommends cutting patches or pills in half and tapering down over two months — either half a dose a day or even a full dose one day and a half dose the next, for a couple of weeks. If you start getting flushes again, go back up to a full dose.

My suggestion is to wean off the patches in winter. In summer you're just asking for trouble — it will be hard to tell whether the hot flushes have come back or you're just hot.

What is the difference between HRT and 'the pill'?

Both use oestrogen and progestogen but HRT is a much lower dose so cannot be relied on for contraception. Given that during perimeno-pause one in three cycles (roughly) are ovulatory, do not rely on HRT alone to prevent a pregnancy. 'The forties is a peak age for unplanned pregnancies, with a high rate of twins,' Professor Bronwyn Stuckey told me. 'The high drive from the pituitary gland often causes the maturation of two eggs.' In fact, you can ovulate twice in a cycle, so you really need to take contraception seriously.

You can safely 'skip periods' on the pill but many women choose to have a break from the pill during which time they take sugar pills and have a bleed every month. The pill can be used to solve both hot flushes and the need for contraception for women under 50 during perimenopause. After age 50, currently, doctors don't like the higher doses of hormones in the pill but some, albeit not many, women are still fertile. So if you're over 50 but still having periods, we'd take you off the pill. If you get symptoms of menopause, we'd switch you to HRT for management of any menopause symptoms. Separately we'd ensure you have additional contraception — for example, a progesterone-containing IUD or condoms.

After menopause you don't need contraception anymore and we wouldn't recommend the pill, so you'd be switched to HRT if you needed it. How would we know if you still needed it? There's no hard science on this but I would tend to take you off the pill (in winter!) when you hit 50 and see how you go.

What if my doctor won't prescribe me HRT?

This is *really* hard. I asked all of the experts and we came to the same conclusion: you might need to change doctors. The Menopause Societies in each jurisdiction (Australia, Britain, Europe, North America) have websites with 'find a doctor' menus. Doctors who join the Menopause Societies have an interest in menopause and that means they are well informed about HRT.

But if you like your GP and don't want to change, or there is no doctor near you with that special interest, you need to advocate on your own behalf. Perhaps take this book with you. Or simply suggest your doctor takes a look at the guidelines coming from their national Menopause Society and ask for the HRT you deserve.

What are bio-identical hormones?

When you have a condition that affects 75 per cent of women and lasts for an average of 7.4 years, and the market leader (HRT) loses 80 per cent of its market share, savvy businesspeople spot opportunities. Since 2002 we have seen the rise and rise of businesses ranging from well-meaning placebo peddlers to full-on multi-million dollar companies scrambling to own the space. I call them the charlatans in the abyss.

In Australia, where I practise, there are celebrities setting up entire online shopping malls of vitamins and other supplements for menopausal women (most of which will do maximum harm to your wallet but not much else). And then there are the so-called 'bio-identical hormone' behemoths. These are touted as 'natural' and 'safe' — claims they can make because they're not regulated. Whoever coined the 'bio-identical' marketing phrase should get a medal for ingenious manipulation of the English language. Because bio-identical sounds clean and natural and safe; and yet, they're just hormones.

These hormone treatments are custom-made at a compounding pharmacy according to a doctor's prescription. Mind you, these might be opportunistically savvy doctors, who recognise both the patient demand and the absence of trust in traditional HRT therapies. But they are hormones, just like HRT. There is no difference between the ingredients per se and the ones I would prescribe you in my GP surgery. For example, oestrogens in bio-identical products are oestradiols — they are just made from a plant chemical extracted from yams and soy rather than the urine of pregnant mares. They are also available as products on prescription from your doctor, and are not unique to the bio-identical hormones. I tend to prescribe oestradiol and never prescribe conjugated equine oestrogen (CEE). Bio-identical progesterone is simply progesterone: it's micronised (finely ground) in the laboratory for better absorption in the body. I love it and use it often for my patients. But I *only* love it when I know what's in it — when it is made under strict supervision by a reputable source.

The main differences between these bio-identical hormones and what your local doctor would prescribe is the level of supervision during the manufacturing process, the price (they're much more expensive than prescription HRT) and the way the hormone is delivered (for example, troches or lozenges that aren't routinely available for prescription medication).

When a regulator, such as the TGA in Australia or the FDA in the US, approves a drug, the drug company then has to report any side effects they are informed of. They then *must*, by law, prominently mention these side effects in the product's package insert. Pharmacies that compound hormones have no such obligations. This has perpetuated the myth that compounded hormones are safer. They're not.

During the manufacturing process, TGA- and FDA-registered factories are audited for cleanliness and accuracy of the product description. If your product is labelled as 50mg of an ingredient but doesn't contain that, there are severe penalties.

Why are my friends taking bio-identical hormones?

With doctors handling the menopause conversation so poorly and in an atmosphere of fear, I'm not surprised that bio-identical hormone businesses have thrived. Yesterday I saw not one but four patients who are taking these products! They hadn't even thought to have the HRT conversation with me. The path for the public, bypassing their GP and going directly to the bio-identical route, is partially helped along by celebrity endorsers such as Oprah who famously declared that 'after one day on bio-identical estrogen, I felt the veil lift'.

The industry of compounding pharmacy surged after the WHI's early shutdown. Women, who were either afraid of 'Big Pharma' HRT or whose doctors wouldn't give it to them, were desperate for some relief. Studies in the US suggest that, of women using some form of HRT, 35 per cent take the bio-identical variety. The pharmacies that supply the bio-identical hormones are set for a significant financial upside. A recent survey of compounding pharmacies found that they're getting set for a projected growth of between 5 and 25 per cent over the next two years!

Aren't they tested?

The whole bio-identical hormone field is based only very loosely on science. Many of my patients show me the long list of expensive blood or saliva tests that have been ordered for them by the doctors they consult either in person, on the end of the phone or online. The special tests are ordered because the treatments are apparently 'individually tailored' to your blood needs. Just to be clear: these tests are nonsense. There's no evidence that your blood levels predict the dose of hormone you need, and these tests are roundly rejected by experts on the basis of lack of evidence.

Bio-identical hormone treatments come as pellets, lozenges, pessaries, troches or creams. Some of these formulations have poor absorption into the body. For example, there is no evidence that either progesterone troches or progesterone creams can protect your endometrium, which is why conventional doctors don't prescribe them.

Oestrogen delivered by troches and many creams and gels are absorbed rapidly, reaching a peak concentration in the bloodstream within one hour, then rapidly dropping back to baseline within about six hours.

I think it's worth mentioning the hormone 'pellet' here. It is a tiny implant of oestrogen and testosterone that is inserted by one of these doctors just under the skin of the buttocks or belly. It slowly releases the two hormones into the body for around six months or so. This is not without risks and, while pellets used to be very popular, the drug companies who were manufacturing them pulled up stumps in 2012. The reason for this decision was that hormone levels from pellets are unpredictable and can stay high for years, even after they have been removed. They are now compounded by pharmacists, without oversight, in exactly the same way as all bio-identical hormones.

One potential risk from super-high levels of hormones is tachyphylaxis, when the pellet releases its hormones too rapidly for your body. These super-high oestrogen doses seem to bring on an early return to hot flushes. But, if we simply replace the pellets when hot flushes return, without measuring your oestrogen levels, you can end up with a major problem.

Experts advise that the implants should be replaced *only* when oestrogen levels fall in your blood.

I saw a patient of mine who had disappeared for a while after I suggested she was entering premature menopause (sadly, it happened for her at age 30). She had gone to a local GP who was prescribing her bio-identical hormones. She had been sucking on troches and using 'natural' creams because she was told HRT would be dangerous for her. When I saw her she had picked up severe osteoporosis and menopausal bleeding. Her dosing on progesterone was completely ineffective, because you can't absorb much progesterone from troches, and the oestrogen was inappropriate for her bone needs. I now have a specialist trying to sort her out.

The North American Menopause Society has this as their position statement: 'Compounded bio-identical HT should be avoided, given concerns about safety, including the possibility of overdosing or under-dosing, lack of efficacy and safety studies, and lack of a label providing risks.'

HRT
THE BOTTOM LINE

HRT is hands down the best way to stop hot flushes and the vaginal and urinary symptoms of menopause; it includes bone strengthening for free.

For women who start HRT within 10 years of menopause, benefits are both short-term (for hot flushes and sexual function) and long-term (for bone health and coronary risk reduction).

We prescribe combination HRT if you have an intact uterus.

Start HRT sooner rather than later and ideally before age 60.

You should have a screening mammogram every two years (on or off HRT) from age 50.

To reduce your risk of breast cancer, get into a healthy weight range, do some exercise and don't drink wine every night.

The International Menopause Society clearly states: 'Healthy women younger than 60 years should not be unduly concerned about the safety profile of HRT. New data and re-analyses of older studies by women's age show that, for most women, the potential benefits of HRT given for a clear indication are many and the risks are few when initiated within a few years of menopause.'

CHAPTER 2

MEET YOUR HORMONES

We can't start to talk about menopause and perimenopause without describing your hormones and their actions. I'm going to take a bit of a sprint through these and give you some definitions.

Menopause marks the effective end-of-production of one of your hormone mega-factories, your ovaries. They have, hopefully, served you well up to this stage, giving you fertility and producing the hormones that help keep you youthful and healthy. Technically, the day of the start of your menopause is 12 months since the first day of your last period. The average age of natural menopause in Western societies is 51 (one to two years earlier for smokers) although the range is huge. Hitting menopause anywhere between 45 and 58 is pretty normal. It does mean that you can expect to live *at least* a third of your life as a postmenopausal woman.

Until that day, you're technically still in perimenopause. Perimenopause ('menopause transition') is defined by the World Health Organization and the North American Menopause Society as the two to eight years preceding menopause and one year following your final period.

What does perimenopause look like? Well, in 10 per cent of women it looks like nothing. Normal life . . . and then one day you realise it's been a year since your last period; so, you've hit menopause with no symptoms at all. Ninety per cent of us get some symptoms, from hot flushes (up to 75 per cent of women) to heavy periods (25 per cent of us), unpredictable irregular periods, vaginal dryness, insomnia, mood problems, exhaustion, low libido and incontinence. Fun? Yeah, right.

What do my ovaries do?

In every typical premenopausal 28-day cycle, an amazing and mysterious miracle takes place: one of your millions of sleepy immature eggs is selected as 'egg of the month'. Under the steady influence of follicle-stimulating hormone (FSH) released by the pituitary gland in the brain, the egg begins to grow inside its follicle or bubble. When the follicle reaches a certain size, it triggers the same pituitary to send in a surge of luteinising hormone (LH). LH tells your follicle to go ahead and release the egg, which heads off down the fallopian tube, hopefully to meet the sperm of her dreams and turn into a baby.

What is left of the follicle is now called a corpus luteum. Along with the name change comes a function change. The corpus luteum produces stacks of progesterone and a more moderate amount of oestrogen; these hormones are essential for the health of the embryo. Assuming the egg didn't meet her Casanova sperm and get fertilised, the corpus luteum eventually fades and, with it, your oestrogen and progesterone levels. Once they are low enough, your uterus can no longer hold on to its lining, which starts to break down and come out as a period. Once you are through menopause, your ovaries no longer release an egg of any sort. Your fertility is over.

Let's take a look at the hormones your ovaries make until menopause, and the effects they have on your body.

Oestrogen

The word oestrogen really refers to a group of hormones: oestrone (E1); oestradiol (E2); and oestriol (E3), plus 50 lesser-known and probably less-relevant hormones. Oestradiol is the most common, the strongest and the most well studied of the oestrogens. Oestrone is weaker than oestradiol and is the more common oestrogen seen in postmenopausal women. Oestriol is the weakest oestrogen of all and is a major player during pregnancy, so we won't discuss it here. The body can easily switch one into any of the others at any time. They're all made in the ovaries out of cholesterol, but small amounts are also made from adrenal sex hormones (see below) and fat cells.

Oestrogen has a number of roles:

- It is the major player when it comes to puberty.

- It controls the menstrual cycle. Under oestrogen's steady influence, the uterus grows stronger, the lining of the uterus grows thicker and the vagina walls become thicker and moister.

- Oestrogen stimulates the brain, which can be great for thinking and memory, but at its extremes can make you feel anxious, agitated and even cause migraines and fits.

- It makes your liver make more HDL, the good cholesterol, and less LDL, the bad cholesterol.

- It can control your weight inasmuch as your fat cells also have oestrogen receptors, and oestrogen tells your body to deposit more fat in the girly spots — thighs, buttocks and breasts — and less on the tummy.

- The skin has oestrogen receptors, too, and is plumper when there's more oestrogen around.

- There are oestrogen receptors on your bone cells, and oestrogen stops bone loss, which, in effect, keeps the bones strong (fending off osteoporosis).

- Oestrogen increases the blood's ability to clot.

- In the gastrointestinal tract, oestrogen slows down the bowel's movements but increases production of bile from the gall bladder to help you break down fats.

- It tells the kidneys to retain fluid and salt, causing swelling of the hands, feet and sometimes the breasts.

- Oestrogen improves the health and tone of your entire urinary tract, helping you defend against infections.

- It boosts your production of sex hormone-binding globulin (SHBG). This protein binds your androgens (see page 45) in the bloodstream, making them less active.

We now know that cells in almost every system in the body have some oestrogen receptors and are affected by our hormonal cycle.

Many of the symptoms of both menopause and perimenopause come from declining oestrogen levels. As your ovaries start aging and running out of puff, they produce less oestrogen. But there is still oestrogen in the body, coming more from other sources. The first of the non-ovarian sources is the, albeit shrinking, pool of adrenal androgen precursors such as DHEA and androsteniedione (see pages 47–8). The second and equally important source of non-ovarian oestrogen is an enzyme, aromatase. As you get older, your fat starts producing more aromatase, which converts testosterone to oestrogens. Aromatase is one of the key targets of medication for oestrogen-fuelled breast cancer in postmenopausal women.

Oestrogen levels basically plummet after menopause when the ovaries stop working altogether. But during perimenopause, the ovaries have big oestrogen production days and lower days, with a seesaw kind of pattern to oestrogen levels.

Progesterone

This is your second major female hormone, produced by your ovaries. The ovarian follicle is the little bubble that housed the egg before it was released by the ovary. After it has released its precious egg into the fallopian tube, in the hope of its being fertilised, the ruptured follicle becomes a corpus luteum and starts spitting out progesterone; 97 per cent of your progesterone is made in this way and the remaining 3 per cent is made by the adrenal glands. Because you stop ovulating before you reach full menopause, your progesterone levels fall before your oestrogen levels. Each month is different in perimenopause — while some months might be low progesterone months, others might be reasonable.

Like oestrogen receptors, progesterone receptors are found all over the body. Progesterone has a number of actions:

- Progesterone makes the endometrium more compact and stops it from overgrowing.

- Progesterone thickens the mucus in the cervix, making it impenetrable to sperm.

- It is a natural nerve-cell calmer, even a sedative for your brain.

- It makes you hungry.

- It is an anti-inflammatory hormone and turns down your immune system.

- It counters oestrogen's role as a fluid retainer by having a mildly diuretic effect on your kidneys.

Androgens, or male hormones

Some women are surprised to hear that we have lots of male hormones, or androgens, in our bodies. It's just that women's levels are only 5 to 10 per cent of men's levels. Androgens, including testosterone, are important in women's health. Roughly half of your male sex hormones are made by your ovaries and the rest by your adrenal glands, via precursor hormones. The adrenal glands basically make a pool of male sex steroids, all of which can be converted into other hormones, and some of which are active themselves.

Androgens have a number of actions in women:

- They increase the oil (or sebum) production of your skin and hair. In excess, they give you oily skin and acne.

- They increase the production of that wiry, coarse pubic and underarm 'terminal' hair. Excess testosterone in women can be responsible for hair in unwanted places (and all of us have some): your legs, the snail trail from belly button to the pubic region, around your nipples and on the chin and upper lip. And, in some women, you can get those thick coarse hairs in other places such as the chest and tummy, lower back, neck and cheeks.

- Androgens increase hair loss from the scalp, especially the very top of the head.

- They probably increase libido and the degree of sexual arousal.

- They increase muscle mass and bone density.

- They increase water and sodium reabsorption from the kidneys, putting up your blood pressure.

- They increase attention, memory and spatial ability.

Because it's a steroid hormone, most of the testosterone in the bloodstream is transported around attached to the carrier protein SHBG, which we met earlier.

As you age, your androgen levels tend to fall off along with your oestrogen and progesterone. But the pattern is different. During perimenopause, your androgen levels go up, and then after menopause they decline slowly. This sets up a situation where there can be an imbalance of oestrogen and androgens, making the androgens relatively more dominant. This all happens because, for some bizarre reason, the ovaries retain the ability to make androgen for years after menopause, despite the fact that they are no longer able to crank out oestrogen and progesterone. And the adrenals don't shut down for ages after menopause, so you have this circulating pool of precursor androgens.

In the vast majority of women, this relatively high testosterone level doesn't give you acne, a deep voice and greasy hair. Chin hairs are another story; they're *very* common from perimenopause on (see Chapter 9, Make me look like Helen Mirren). But it does increase your risk of high blood pressure and heart disease after menopause.

Pregnenolone

Pregnenolone is actually a precursor form of almost all steroid hormones, such as oestrogen, progesterone and testosterone. It also has direct effects on the brain. It inhibits the neurotransmitter GABA, which is your brain's natural built-in sedative. GABA slows down nerve firing in the brain, combatting anxiety and stress. It also makes you sleepy. More pregnenolone = less

GABA = MORE brain firing! It's a 'wake up and start thinking' hormone! Certainly in Petri dishes and in rats, pregnenolone also stimulates the growth of new brain cells, especially in the hippocampus (that enhances memory).

It tends to decline over time, just as a result of normal aging. Research is underway as to whether pregnenolone itself could be used to combat age-related memory loss and poorer brain function. There have been conflicting results from studies in mice, and the jury is still out as to whether it is worthwhile. Certainly lots of people report feeling sharper while taking it, although the experts I chatted to when researching this book were very sceptical. Probably the most important thing to know about pregnenolone is that if you Google menopause, it's a term that will come up repeatedly — and almost everything you read about it will be BS.

DHEA

This is one of the adrenal androgens that pregnenolone turns into. DHEA hormones are like a big pool of highly flexible sex hormones that can easily be converted to either oestrogen or testosterone in the tissues. Unlike pregnenolone, DHEA itself doesn't do anything to your cells. No specific DHEA receptor has ever been identified, but what we do know is that DHEA is the precursor for 100 per cent of circulating androgens and oestrogens in postmenopausal women after the ovaries have run out of steam. So, without it, your hormone levels will fall through the floor.

You really start producing lots of DHEA at around six to eight years of age. Your blood levels of DHEA peak somewhere between the age of 20 and 30, and after that they slowly but steadily decline. By the time you hit 80 years of age, your blood levels of DHEA are only 10 to 20 per cent of their peak levels.

We know from studies that, if you have blood levels of DHEA below the tenth percentile, you definitely have a higher chance of having sexual problems both before and after you start menopause. Other studies have linked low blood levels of DHEA with a lower (general) feeling of wellbeing in women. Certainly many of the anti-aging specialists, especially in the US, believe that supplementing DHEA may have anti-aging effects. But studies have had mixed results. Critics point out that stress and chronic illness, both of which definitely snuff out your libido, also suppress your DHEA levels. Maybe the low DHEA doesn't cause the sexual problems, but rather both low DHEA and low libido are symptoms of stress, so treating one will, at best, only give you a placebo effect. Plus, we don't know whether they can contribute to breast cancer in women (and prostate cancer in men).

Androstenedione

This is another reserve hormone that is a precursor to both oestrogen and testosterone. It is made by a chemical reaction altering DHEA. There are two sources of androstenedione in the body: the first is in the adrenal gland, like your DHEA; the rest is made by the ovaries.

Your androstenedione levels start to rise in the lead up to puberty, mainly coming from the maturing adrenal glands. But they only reach adult levels around age 18. Then they start to fall and by menopause they're very low again.

What happens to all these hormones during perimenopause and menopause?

I want to start by saying that this area is poorly understood, including by doctors. It wasn't until I was going through perimenopause myself that I got my teeth into the research and started hounding the experts.

The easy part to understand is actual menopause. By now your follicles have completely stopped working and practically no oestrogen is being made from your ovaries. A small amount of oestrogen will come from your fat (via aromatase, the enzyme that sits in fat cells and converts testosterone to oestrogen). And a small amount comes from the adrenal precursor hormones. But your oestrogen has pretty much flatlined.

It's perimenopause, the era I like to call hormone hell, that has everyone befuddled.

The PENN-5 staging system (devised by the University of Pennsylvania) divides perimenopause into five stages: premenopausal (regular menstrual cycles of 21–35 days); late premenopausal (one change in cycle length of at least seven days); early menopause transition (at least two cycles with cycle length changes of at least seven days); late transition (greater than or equal to three months of no periods); and postmenopausal (greater than or equal to 12 months of no periods).

While menopause and perimenopause are often thrown in together, hormonally they are as different as chalk and cheese. We know that progesterone does indeed start a steady decline from perimenopause. This decline starts way before your periods even start to become erratic. It finally falls close to zero as you hit menopause. During perimenopause, you start ovulating less often and the ovulations you do have don't give you a nice, well-functioning corpus luteum, so your ovaries simply can't make progesterone like they used to.

Old-school thinking was that oestrogen does the same thing: a slow decline. We now know that the picture is far more complex. Many studies have shown that, in fact, during perimenopause your oestrogen fluctuates up and down like a yoyo. This is because, as your ovaries are getting a little weaker and just cranking out less oestrogen generally, your pituitary gland in your brain leaps into gear and starts pushing out FSH. These slightly aging ovaries will move between sluggishly ignoring the FSH, to having a massive response and pushing out stacks of oestrogen. So, you can oscillate between low oestrogen and excessive oestrogen month to month, week to week, even day to day.

In the final stages of perimenopause, particularly in the one to two years prior to your final period, your oestrogen levels finally do decline and you get less episodes of the excess oestrogen. Plus your androgens are doing a last bizarre surge before true menopause starts. All of which leaves you in hormone hell. On days when you get excess oestrogen and lack of progesterone, you'll enjoy insomnia, anxiety, breast tenderness and swelling. The next day your oestrogen levels might fall, so you may get hot flushes from oestrogen withdrawal. Blood hormone level tests at this time are utterly useless, because the levels one day bear no relation to the levels the next day or the next week.

It's a difficult time for fertility too. The high levels of FSH can see women ovulate not once but twice. So, in terms of fertility, you kind of lurch between very low fertility, and extreme excess fertility with a high risk of twins. And if you've had anxiety or depression before, watch out. You hit peak emotional roller-coaster around the time of your menopause transition.

YOUR HORMONES
THE BOTTOM LINE

There are lots of them and they're complicated.

Perimenopause sees your hormones waxing and waning and definitely out of proportion with each other, leaving most women feeling pretty sub-optimal.

Menopause sees the oestrogen and progesterone output of your ovaries decline to zero.

Male androgen hormones have their own timing agenda, lasting far longer than oestrogen and progesterone in most women.

CHAPTER 3

BAPTISM BY FIRE

You're sitting in a meeting. Let's say it's a *really* important meeting. Then you start to feel a clammy heat in your chest, as if perhaps someone has started burning you at the stake without you noticing. Now it's spreading up your neck, and there it goes . . . to your face. You know you've turned beetroot red beneath the foundation you layered on to hide just such a moment. Beads of sweat gather between your breasts, on the back of your neck, through your scalp and across your lip. You're torn between the unbearable need to rip off your jacket or perhaps find a bucket of cold water, and needing to look and sound calm, controlled and professional. And then it's gone, followed by a nice chill — there's nothing like cooling sweat in an intensely air-conditioned meeting room.

At their extreme, hot flushes can happen every hour, including right through the night, meaning decent sleep becomes a dim memory. They can make you grumpy and fearful — when is the next one coming? Given that they are more likely to happen and be at their worst during times of stress, this is a vicious catch 22.

The stats are not on your side. A massive 75 per cent of women get hot flushes; so, if you don't, consider yourself very lucky. Typically, they look like a sudden wave of heat. They can come packaged up with sweating, reddening of the skin and rapid heartbeat. They usually last three to four minutes, but *can* range from one to 60 minutes.

They can happen at any time of day or night. They can be triggered by embarrassment, sudden temperature change, stress, alcohol, caffeine (or any warm drink for that matter). Or they can happen for no reason at all. And they are often very, very distressing.

A variation on the theme is the night sweat. These are hot flushes that come on at night and disturb your sleep. It can take you half an hour to cool down enough after a flush to go back to sleep, at which point you can have another one. It's like having a newborn again, but worse. You might be up five or six times a night, throwing off the covers and drenched pyjamas, then feeling cold and having to put on fresh ones. Your sleep is shot and after a while that takes a toll on your physical and mental health.

If this isn't ringing true for you, you might be someone whose hot flushes are simply milder. Many women just run hotter: no dramatic beet-root-red faces but just a general feeling of being heat intolerant. You might be more prone to developing an unladylike glow and damp underarm patch, having to wear a light shirt, or being the pain in the neck at work who needs the air conditioning set to 15 degrees when everyone else is shivering in a sweater. Or you might just feel hot and sweaty in bed so that a full night's sleep is impossible.

Either way, hot flushes can range from annoying to horrific.

What causes my hot flushes?

I can tell you that the answer, today anyway, is that we don't know the full story. But we know bits of it. For example, we know that the flushes come from *falling* (but not necessarily low) levels of oestrogen. We know this because they come on around menopause and because giving women oestrogen in the form of HRT usually fixes them. Plus, we know that menopausal and perimenopausal women with hot flushes don't have lower levels of oestrogen in their blood, urine or even their vaginas than those of women at the same stage of life without hot flushes. So we know it is not about low levels of oestrogen per se. And, finally, pre-pubertal girls have very low oestrogen levels but they don't get hot flushes.

The flushes themselves are triggered by tiny elevations in core body temperature. It seems women who get hot flushes have a smaller 'thermo-neutral zone' — that's the comfort range between upper (sweating) and lower (shivering) temperature thresholds. So that, with only minor changes in body temperature, the body perceives a major change and responds by going to extreme measures to cool you down — sweating and sending heat to the skin to seep out.

We know this involves activation of the sympathetic nervous system via the hypothalamus. The latest research suggests that there are neurons or nerve cells in the hypothalamus that detect changes in temperature and make bodily adjustments (for example, shivering to increase the body temperature, or sweating and opening blood vessels to divert blood to the skin so that heat can be lost through the skin). These neurons seem to be *linked* to the neurons in the hypothalamus that detect falling oestrogen levels in the blood, so that small falls in oestrogen can trigger a heat reaction inside the hypothalamus.

In response, the body does actually get hotter and yet it's not the way it often feels. For example, we know that when you measure body tempera-ture, the biggest temperature jumps are found in the fingers and toes! And yet you feel the flushing in the face, neck and chest (despite the fact that the actual temperature increase in these areas is only about 1 degree C). Plus the increase in temperature by measurement lasts for ages after the feeling of the hot flush has disappeared.

A fairly recently discovered brain chemical called neurokinin B (NKB) seems to play a crucial role. Both animal and human trials have shown that increased levels of NKB might trigger hot flushes. This is relevant because *decreasing* NKB could then be a cure for hot flushes.

There are things that make hot flushes worse. Smoking, lack of physical activity, lower socio-economic status, negative mood and negative atti-tudes towards menopause have all been linked in studies to worse hot flushes. Make of that what you will! And there could be racial or cultural factors, too. The numbers I have been quoting are predominantly for white women in North America, Europe and Australia. Women in Asia are much less likely to report hot flushes as a concern. But, to complicate things further, there may be other biological, cultural or psychological factors at play. According to one study, Indian women in India are less than half as likely to report hot flushes as being a primary concern, than Indian women who have migrated to England. And for those who migrated to England? Well, they were just as likely as native European women to experience hot flushes.

I'm personally fascinated by family history and hot flushes. I suspect that if your mum had them, you're more likely to cop them, too. But it turns out that nobody has ever done a study, so we have no idea whether genes play a role.

How long will I have hot flushes?

The news is good or bad, depending on how you view it. In most cases, time is a great healer and if you wait them out they almost always go away. The problem is, it is often a long wait. On average, hot flushes last for 7.4 years. But US researchers found that women who started getting hot flushes during perimenopause — before their final period — have hot flushes that tend to last longer. Their hot flushes last for an average of 11.8 years and they are termed the 'super flushers'. By contrast, if the flushes don't start until women are established in menopause, the flushes generally last around five to seven years. And then there are the long-term flushers. Studies from Australia and the US find that 42 per cent of women aged 60–65 still get hot flushes. According to Professor John Eden, Head of the Sydney Menopause Centre at the Royal Hospital for Women, one in eight women who get flushes, flush forever. Ouch.

Many of my patients tell me they are not bothered by their flushes and feel no need to try to fix them. That's great, but I do suspect some women say that because they're so fearful of HRT, they're worried I'll grab a prescription pad and force them into what they see as a dangerous solution. I'm no zealot for any particular therapy, but I am a zealot for your empowerment to make choices from the greatest range of beneficial options. I'm most interested in simply alleviating your symptoms. If the flushes seriously don't bother you, that's brilliant. But, given the number of home remedies submitted to *Medicine or Myth?* for hot flushes, and the amount written online, I think they bother a *lot* of women. Evidence is that, of the 75 per cent of us who get them, a third have them at severe levels. And only a third get them 'mildly'. So whether they last three years or twenty, we need a solution.

What could I try first?

I'm going to whiz through these because you've probably already tried most of them … and I'm guessing they haven't worked adequately or you wouldn't be here.

* Dress in layers.
* Wear sleeveless tops.
* Wear natural fibres.
* Avoid jumpers — too hard to take off quickly! Cardigans are a total fashion statement.
* Carry a fan in your bag.
* Put layers on your bed so you can keep a sheet on and throw off the duvet.
* Two separate duvets is a good option if your partner is being disturbed by your night-time temperature changes.
* Have a fan and/or air conditioning in the bedroom.
* Put a cold pack under your pillow (or try a cooling pillow).
* Avoid your known triggers.

If you know what your triggers are, you can avoid them or at least have on hand strategies to help. Yours might be spicy foods, alcohol, stress or changes in temperatures. Lots of my patients tell me a hot shower almost always leads to disaster; so, take two icepacks from the freezer into the bathroom with you and shove one under each armpit when you step out of the shower.

What lifestyle measures are worth pursuing?

Lose weight

Higher BMI (body mass index) is definitely linked to more and worse hot flushes. In fact, in one study, once your BMI got over 25, your risk of having hot flushes went up. Those with a BMI of 25 were 1.7 times more likely to have hot flushes than those with a BMI of less than 22. The higher your BMI, the worse the flushing. I've always found this strange because, as I explained in Chapter 2, aromatase converts androstenedione to oestrogen. Meaning, fatter people have higher oestrogen levels, so they should have *fewer* hot flushes, right?

It seems instead that the extra 'insulation' in the body somehow narrows the 'thermoneutral zone' to make you more susceptible to the unwanted effects of even slight changes in temperature.

Weirdly, not many studies have been done to assess the role of weight loss in controlling menopausal hot flushes. But when you look at the small studies that *have* been done, the North American Menopause Society (NAMS) says there's enough evidence to recommend weight loss as a tool to reduce the burden of hot flushes. (See Chapter 7, Where did my waistline go?)

Stop smoking

Lots of studies find that smokers get more hot flushes than non-smokers, especially during perimenopause — although we don't know for sure why. And yet not one study has been done to assess whether giving up smoking will help with your hot flushes. I think that's because every doctor alive will advise you to stop smoking and no study is going to change that, regardless of the outcome. So I'll just join the throng: seriously, quit.

Have a glass of wine (or vodka or beer, if that's your thing)

That's not a joke. Studies show that *light* alcohol consumption is associated with lower odds of suffering hot flushes than never drinking alcohol. This is true for menopause and perimenopause. We have absolutely no idea why this might be, although one theory that has been raised is that wine can increase your blood-glucose levels. Other studies have shown slightly higher blood-glucose levels can reduce the severity of hot flushes. Just a theory for now!

Use cooling mattresses and pillows

So don't look for the studies: the info I bring you comes from the University of my Girlfriends. What I have been able to glean is this: you can buy actual mattress 'toppers' that are plush extra cushioning for comfort. It seems that some toppers are advertised as also giving good temperature control to cool down your mattress. Toppers that 'sleep cool' without altering the temperature of the bed are known as 'passive cooling toppers' and tend to be made from materials such as latex or gel-infused foam. You can also buy 'active cooling toppers', which actually create colder sleep surfaces by using built-in components, such as fans or water tanks. Ditto, pillows for women who have partners who don't want to be cooled down at night. I've been told you can also have a king bed with two separate king single mattresses on it — then you have your own single mattress cooler and your partner doesn't freeze.

These are very big hits with my buddies and also with my 25-year-old son, who lives life at a high temperature! Night-time heat was interfering with his sleep, so that was a birthday present that went down a treat.

Try mind-based therapies

Don't knock it: these can work if you can get past your scepticism. Randomised, double-blind, controlled trials have shown that a cognitive behavioural therapy (CBT) based treatment, combining relaxation and sleep strategies with learning to take a more positive, healthy approach to menopause's many challenges, was a winning strategy. It significantly reduced the women's ratings of the impact of their hot flushes (although interestingly, not the amount). Specifically, targeting negative thoughts about hot flushes ('everyone's looking at me'), feeling you've lost control ('there's nothing I can do' or 'I'll never get back to sleep'), and reactions to hot flushes such as avoiding socialising, as well as stress, can all yield dividends. As a result, NAMS recommends mind-based approaches.

On the other hand, after a ton of studies, the jury is in and, sadly, studies have found that yoga and other exercise, breathing exercises and, acupuncture are all fairly useless for hot flushes. But, especially in the case of yoga and other exercise, they're so packed with health benefits that we still want you to do them. We just can't in good faith tell you they'll reduce your hot flushes.

The evidence for relaxation, calibration of neural oscillations (a very odd-sounding brain-training technique) and chiropractic treatment is very flaky. NAMS said in their position statement that these therapies are unlikely to help.

What about the placebo effect?

Before I dive into the medical alternatives available for managing hot flushes, I have to talk about the placebo effect (the improvement that someone experiences, particularly in areas of sensation such as pain or discomfort, when taking what they think is a 'remedy' but which actually has no possible objective mechanism to address the underlying sensation). A properly controlled trial will include a placebo arm, in order to compare the actual (perceived + medical) effects of the remedy with the benefits that exist only in the perception of the person being treated. In studies of hot flushes, the placebo effect can be very high.

It's difficult to make sense of what this means. Is the discomfort 'real' or is it just 'in your head'. The reality is that pain and sensation is a complex area that we don't fully understand. And, while attitude has a big impact on the sensation of discomfort, so, too, do effective remedies. So more than anywhere, this is where your personal views and experiences are just as valid as 'the science'.

NAMS ran an analysis across all trials of alternative medicines and medications that weren't actually HRT and found that when it comes to hot flushes, there is a staggering placebo improvement rate of between 20 and 60 per cent. It is the more anxious women who have the highest response to placebo — and I think it's good to keep that in mind when reading through the evidence behind some of the studies that support alternative treatments.

Something else to keep in mind when evaluating a treatment for hot flushes is this: studies have found that neither the number of flushes, nor the length of flushes, necessarily determines how much they worry a woman. But they're easy to measure. So a treatment might decrease the number of flushes by 50 per cent and still not make the woman feel any better. But another treatment might reduce the number of flushes by only one a day and yet give enormous relief. So, when choosing a treatment for hot flushes, quality is more important than quantity.

My flushes are still interfering with my quality of life: what could I take?

The real concern I have in addressing this section is the fear and bullshit that is foisted on us. From the original distortion of the HRT trial findings, to charlatans pushing ineffective and potentially harmful remedies, there are many 'bad actors' in this space.

My job is to sift through the misconceptions and point out potential harms associated with the available remedies, to help you and your health-care professional make the best choice for you. So let's dive in.

HRT

I have written in detail about HRT and its effect on menopause symptoms, including and especially hot flushes. Just to recap, it is *the most* effective method we have to nix hot flushes. Several studies have shown that HRT fixes hot flushes in up to 98 per cent of women.

Evidence suggests that HRT is having a bit of a renaissance after being wrongly maligned by women and their doctors for so many years. It makes me very happy to see a woman get her sleep back, lose the embarrassing and uncomfortable flushes, maybe get back her libido and enjoyment of sex, and see her mood improve. But, as we've discussed, many women have very different experiences when approaching their doctors about menopausal symptoms. One of the experts I approached for this book told me she went to her GP and asked specifically for HRT for her hot flushes and was refused. It was too dangerous, she was told. She switched GPs and got a prescription pronto. 'I've never looked back,' she told me. As a busy clinician and academic, she wasn't about to walk away from her job because of impossible menopause symptoms. Especially when she knew there was such an effective treatment out there.

But I worry about women who just take the 'no HRT' mantra at face value and don't get another opinion. I worry about women who don't want to be 'difficult' or who feel guilty about asking for a pill for a 'natural phenomenon'. These women end up exhausted, depressed and so uncomfortable from their flushes that it impacts on their work and leisure — they're not getting the menopause experience they could have, if given the right treatment.

I am *not* saying HRT is right for all of us. But if your hot flushes are impacting on your life and you don't have a specific reason not to take it (for example, you have breast cancer *now*), you should have access to treatments that work. And the best is HRT.

Tibolone

Tibolone is a progestogen that's unusual in that it has oestrogen-, progesterone- and androgen-like effects. It is excellent at decreasing hot flushes. It's not as effective as HRT but comes a close second: only 8–14 per cent of women who take Tibolone still get hot flushes. In randomised trials, Tibolone has been shown to not only alleviate hot flushes, but also to improve bone density, to help with various aspects of female sexual function and to have less effects on breast tissue than combined HRT. Tibolone also has a lower rate of breakthrough vaginal bleeding in the first three months of treatment. Its effects on sexual function are partly because it is also partially broken down into testosterone. I have suggested it for use by women with low libido but, to be honest, I have found it to be a bit disappointing. Libido is *so* complex. (See Chapter 4, What the hell happened to my vagina?)

The thing to be aware of with Tibolone is the risk of depression. In studies where it is compared to a placebo, Tibolone is great for mood. But many of the specialists I spoke to have the opposite experience. Tibolone often makes depression worse. Dr Fiona Jane is a specialist women's health

GP, who consults at Jean Hailes for Women's Health in Melbourne and is a Research Fellow in the Women's Health Research Program at Monash University. In her opinion, Tibolone won't usually cause depression but it can make depression a whole lot worse. As a result, she would never prescribe it for women with hot flushes if they also have a history of depression. This is partly due to the ingredients of Tibolone activating the corticosteroid receptors in the brain.

But does Tibolone cause cancer? Results have been mixed. The huge UK Million Women Study found that Tibolone increased the risk of breast cancer more than oestrogen-only therapy, but less than combined HRT. But in the LIFT study, breast cancer risk was lower among women taking Tibolone than those on placebo. By the way, the LIFT trial had to be wound up early because they found an increased risk of stroke. Bottom line: if you've had breast cancer before, you can't take Tibolone. At this stage it looks like Tibolone doesn't increase your risk of blood clots. But the LIFT study found a twofold increase risk of stroke. Especially in the first year. That is off a pretty low base though — stroke is rare below the age of 65.

SERM and oestrogen combination, also known as tissue-selective estrogen complex (TSEC)

Selective estrogen receptor modulators (SERM) are drugs that activate some oestrogen receptors in the body and not others. I already mentioned that you can now get a TSEC (Bazedoxifene, a SERM in combination with conjugated oestrogen) in one pill. It works well to reduce hot flushes without needing progestogens, but without any action on breast issue and with a lower risk of vaginal tenderness and vaginal bleeding. The number of studies of TSECs for hot flushes isn't huge and they don't seem to be as effective as HRT, but they're a pretty good alternative. They work well on vaginal tissue, too (See Chapter 4, What the hell happened to my vagina?) and help strengthen bones to prevent osteoporosis. They are slowly becoming more popular as their use increases. I prefer to use them for women who get too sleepy on micronised progesterone and don't want to use it vaginally. It can also be good for women who have a history of depression on the pill. Even though micronised progesterone is a good option for those women, the TSEC can be a nice alternative. It also has lower rates of vaginal breakthrough bleeding and breast pain, so can be useful in those situations.

Antidepressants

I'm including these because they're an important tool for managing flushes in women who have had breast cancer, blood clots or some other condition that rules out HRT. The interest in drugs that increase serotonin in the brain comes because we see an immediate 50 per cent drop in serotonin levels after menopause.

A reasonable number of studies show that these medications work pretty well, although nowhere near as well as HRT. Unless there are red flags, NAMS recommends any of the following three antidepressants for managing hot flushes: Venlafaxine (37.5 to 75mg per day), Paroxetine (12.5 to 25mg per day and now a new 7.5mg dose formulated specifically for hot flushes), or Fluoxetine (20mg per day). I have patients on all of them. If you're on Tamoxifen (a breast-cancer treatment that has oestrogen receptors in it), check that any antidepressant you take is safe to combine with it. Some antidepressants make Tamoxifen less potent, so aren't used.

This group of treatments does have side effects, especially drowsiness, dizziness and constipation. Red flags in medical speak mean that you shouldn't ever use these antidepressants if you are taking certain medications. For example, MAOs (a specific and unusual antidepressant medicine) can sometimes interact adversely with Warfarin (a blood-thinning medication) if used at the same time. Your GP should be across all of this.

Clonidine

This is interesting: it's actually an old-school blood-pressure drug that also works for hot flushes, although side effects include blurred vision, low blood pressure and dopiness. Clonidine appears to widen the 'thermoneutral zone'. Two small placebo-controlled studies found that Clonidine tablets reduced the number of hot flushes by 46 per cent, and Clonidine patches by 80 per cent. Unfortunately, the patches are only available in the US at the moment.

Oxybutynin

This drug is widely used to treat urinary incontinence from an overactive bladder, but was found to be surprisingly effective in the treatment of hot flushes in breast-cancer survivors. This led to a study in women without breast cancer and . . . guess what? Their hot flushes reduced by around 80 per cent. Not as good as HRT, but not bad either. Professor Eden told me that the lower-dose 2.5mg tablet given twice a day has been successful for his patients and has proved relatively free of side effects. It does interact with some medications though, so make sure to discuss these with your doctor and pharmacist.

Gabapentin

This anti-epilepsy drug is also sometimes used for bad nerve pain; it possibly works for hot flushes by direct action on the thermoregulatory centre in the hypothalamus. One downside is that it needs to be taken three times a day. And a nasty side effect from Gabapentin is drowsiness — good at night, terrible during the day. Some people also get dizziness and swelling. Look, it *does* work for hot flushes, but I rarely prescribe it, because when you add up the price, the need to take it three times a day, and the side effects, I just feel there are better options out there.

Pregabalin

Pregabalin is another drug that is designed to reduce nerve pain by suppressing the signals of faulty nerves. Chemically, it is similar to Gabapentin and, for that reason, researchers started looking into it as a possible treatment for hot flushes in menopause. A randomised placebo-controlled trial that involved 163 postmenopausal women was done over a six-week period. It showed that Pregabalin at doses of 75mg twice daily and 150mg twice daily reduced hot flushes by 65 per cent and 71 per cent, respectively, compared to only 50 per cent in the placebo group. Pregabalin is more convenient than Gabapentin, as it's taken twice daily rather than three times. But it's not without its own side effects. Drowsiness and feeling vague are the most commonly reported, but weight gain is a risk at the higher doses. Pregabalin would have to be used 'off label' (meaning, not endorsed by the manufacturers) for hot flushes. But if you can't take HRT, it could be a good option. I'd stick to the 75mg twice daily dose to minimise the side effects.

What about complementary and herbal remedies for hot flushes?

Strap yourself in: there are a ton of these. When we filmed *Medicine or Myth?* we were inundated with 'cures' for hot flushes. Studies show that up to 80 per cent of women will try a non-hormonal treatment for their hot flushes.

I guess it's no surprise. After all, hot flushes are so common and women are really concerned about the safety of HRT. And there are many women who, for medical reasons, can't take HRT. The problem is that the evidence for most of these treatments is pretty weak. Certainly compared to HRT and the other medications I've detailed in the last few pages.

However, the placebo effect is significant when it comes to hot flushes, as we already discussed. Australian menopause expert Professor Rod Baber suggests that with any of the therapies over the next few pages, if you're going to give them a go, give them six weeks maximum. After that, they're unlikely to help and you'll just prolong the financial cost and the misery. You might as well move on and find something that will work.

I am prefacing herbal remedies with three comments:

There is very little evidence for any herbal remedy. However, there is some anecdotal suggestion that in certain circumstances some of the remedies may help.

I've included many of these remedies because they're talked about a lot online, often with close-to-no objective, science-based information. This section aims to give you clarity about some of the remedies you'll find online or peddled by Instagram influencers.

Finally, there are quite a few remedies that fall squarely in the quackery space. I will revert to my Gwyneth rating for these, with zero Gwyneths being reasonable and three Gwyneths being top-ranking pseudoscience BS.

Soy isoflavones

Isoflavones are plant-derived chemicals that can activate some oestrogen receptors in the body. Soybeans and soy products are the richest sources of isoflavones in the human diet. Soy-derived isoflavones include genistein, daidzein, equol and ipriflavone, among others. Many of these compounds are more than 1000 times less active than oestradiol, so a lot of scientists are sceptical about whether they can, on their own, do much for hot flushes. They're interesting chemicals in that they switch on the oestrogen receptors in some tissues, such as bones (good for bone health) and switch off oestrogen receptors in other tissues, such as the lining of the uterus and possibly the breast tissue. So they're being explored as cancer preventers in the women's cancer research space. But the area of hot flushes is a bit less exciting and the trial results of soy isoflavones haven't been that impressive.

There are a couple of reasons. Problem number one is the enormous variation in concentration of these isoflavones in naturally occurring soy. From one batch of tofu to the next, they're not entirely predictable. Problem number two is that some isoflavones, such as genistein, equol and daidzein, require degradation to their active forms by intestinal bacteria in order to become bio-available. They're enormously dependent on the health of your own microbiome, so you can't necessarily eat more tofu to get more isoflavones.

What does this all mean for women wanting to control their hot flushes? Increased dietary soy (from foods such as legumes and tofu) and isoflavone supplements *do* reduce menopause symptoms, but at levels roughly the same as placebo. Let's not diss a totally excellent placebo response. Go for it, if you like — unless you have had breast cancer. We don't have enough safety data to green-light soy in that situation. Neutral on the Gwyneth scale.

Red clover

Red clover has its own isoflavones, too. Lots of studies have shown it to be quite favourable in terms of reducing hot flushes and even helping with vaginal symptoms. However, they were all panned by the Cochrane Collaboration (the doctors who release the highly regarded Cochrane reviews) who found that, on balance, the positive studies were just not very well done. As they pointed out: 'There was a strong placebo effect in most trials with a reduction in frequency ranging from 1 per cent to 59 per cent with placebo.' The same review found no harmful effects. Again, I'm a fan of the effects, whether caused by placebo or otherwise. The downside of red clover is minimal except for the expense. If nothing else works, it might be worth a shot. Zero Gwyneths.

Black cohosh (*Cimicifuga racemosa* or *Actaea racemosa*)

This North American plant has been used for centuries for 'women's ailments' and is the most popular supplement *by far* taken by my patients for treating their hot flushes. Today, black cohosh supplements are made from the plant's roots and rhizomes (underground stems). You can buy the powdered whole herb, liquid extracts and pills.

We don't really know which compounds in black cohosh make it effective. There are heaps of them (none of which I'll name now, in the interests of you not falling asleep). And, like so many plant-based compounds, the ingredients within the plants can't be standardised. From plant to plant — even within different roots of the same plant — there is a huge amount of variability. It's made studying the stuff a bit fraught.

Sadly, objective evidence for black cohosh is practically zero. A 2012 Cochrane review of 16 randomised clinical trials of black cohosh for menopausal symptoms, including hot flushes, night sweats and vaginal dryness, gave a grim report. While there were a couple of good results, they were from the smaller, less scientifically rigorous trials. The two biggest and best trials found no benefit, and worse outcomes for those taking black cohosh than the placebo! Another 2016 review, with a few extra trials included, gave it a big thumbs down.

Original studies blamed black cohosh for liver damage. That hasn't been found in subsequent studies and experts now think it was due to a contaminant. So, if you see a warning on the box, you might not need to worry too much about it; talk it through with your doctor or pharmacist.

Professor Eden tells me he does use black cohosh to augment the effects of Tibolone when the hot flushes aren't quite being controlled but increasing the dose of Tibolone isn't the best option. For example, a woman taking

Tibolone who is feeling better but is still getting some breakthrough hot flushes. Since he gave me this advice, I have been doing likewise and it does help some women so I think it's worth a shot. Remember: six weeks max and then bail out if it isn't working. Zero Gwyneths.

Wild yam cream

Wild yam contains diosgenin, the phytoestrogen. There has been one single trial of this and the results were pretty ordinary. When given as a cream for three months, there were no improvements of menopausal symptoms noted by women, compared with the placebo. On the plus side, in this study there were no side effects reported. However, given the evidence suggests that yam creams are ineffective for menopause and because many contain some contaminants, experts say they should be avoided. Two Gwyneths from me.

Evening primrose oil

Only one study has looked at whether evening primrose oil improves hot flushes. That one study found absolutely no benefit. Unfortunately, evening primrose oil *does* have side effects. It's a no-no for anyone with epilepsy: it lowers the seizure threshold and interferes with the actions of anti-epileptic medication. Other known side effects include diarrhoea and nausea. It gets three Gwyneths from me — save your money.

Flaxseed

This has a similar story to other isoflavones, in that it requires breakdown by gut bacteria to produce very weak oestrogen effects. Back in 2007, a small pilot study of 29 women by researchers at the Mayo Clinic found that consuming 40g of crushed flaxseed a day helped reduce hot flushes. Then the same group went back and did a larger study and found basically no difference between flaxseed and placebo. (Although both groups saw a reduction of menopausal symptoms by 50 per cent — which again makes me love the placebo effect!) There were a lot of side effects in both groups (both had seeds). The increased fibre for the study participants was probably what was behind the diarrhoea, bloating and nausea. Sadly, another no from NAMS, and three Gwyneths from me!

Sage leaf

We were overwhelmed by applicants for *Medicine or Myth?* with remedies for hot flushes — many involving sage leaf or, to be specific, sage-leaf tea. For the show, we commissioned a randomised placebo-controlled trial. Our results were pretty ordinary (30 per cent felt some objective relief, which is slightly below the figures we'd expect for placebo).

There have been a couple of small trials for sage. One Swiss trial without a placebo arm had some incredible results for a sage-leaf tablet taken once a day. The mean number of mild, moderate, severe and very severe flushes decreased by 46 per cent, 62 per cent, 79 per cent, and 100 per cent, respectively, over eight weeks. An Iranian randomised placebo-controlled trial found some pretty good results, too. After eight weeks, the authors said, hot flushes and night sweats were far more reduced in the women who took the sage tablets three times a day than those taking the placebo, even though their hormone levels didn't change. In both trials there were no major side effects and generally sage leaf is found to be very well tolerated, so I'd say it's worth a shot. I tasted sage-leaf tea when we were filming *Medicine or Myth?* and really liked it. So, zero Gwyneths for the taste alone!

Ginseng (*Panax ginseng* or *Panax quinquefolius*)

This remedy appears to have no benefits and plenty of potential harms. No studies have found *Panax ginseng* to have any benefit over placebo for hot flushes. Case reports in medical journals have linked ginseng with bleeding from the vagina, and sore and lumpy breasts. Plus it can't be used with sleeping tablets, such as benzodiazepines, certain antidepressants or anticoagulants; it reduces the effects of immunosuppressive drugs; and it increases the effect of diabetic drugs, so can give some diabetics a hypo event. Another one I'm awarding three Gwyneths.

Maca (*Lepidium meyennii Walp* or *Lepidium peruvianum Chacon*)

Maca is a traditional foodstuff from South America — a cruciferous root grown exclusively in the Peruvian Andes at 4000 to 5000 metres. These rare plants often take on mythical reputations. It turns out that maca does have weak oestrogenic effects, seen in a Petri dish but not actually in humans.

The studies that show some improvement in menopausal symptom scores are pretty shoddy, and maca gets no thumbs up from NAMS. On the plus side, it seems to be pretty safe. I had a bit of a sticky beak online and the doses vary from 200 to 10,000mg per capsule. None of the studies used the same dose, so who knows what the right dose is and if it did anything? Two Gwyneths from me.

Pine bark (Pycnogenol)

Pine bark from the Mediterranean pine (*Pinus pinaster*) is a source of pro-anthocyanidins (also found in grapeseed). Pine bark has only been studied in three randomised controlled trials; the trials were small and not amazingly well conducted but it's looking pretty promising for hot flushes. All three trials used different doses, so finding the right dose is a bit guess-and-check right now. NAMS has called pine bark 'probably safe'. My verdict? Zero Gwyneths — definitely worth a shot.

Pollen extract

We only have one tiny randomised controlled trial for bee pollen, but it did show some improvement in menopausal symptoms. However, on a single study of 53 people, nobody would be game to make a firm recommendation! There are some safety concerns related to pollen allergy. Three Gwyneths if you suffer from allergies!

Licorice root

On a positive note, this has no negative studies. That's because it has no studies at all. Licorice root is a common ingredient in traditional Chinese medicine preparations. Large and long-term doses of licorice can cause dangerous heart rhythms, cardiac arrest and 'pseudoprimary aldosteronism' — a condition that includes high blood pressure, low potassium levels and swelling. I'm giving it three Gwyneths. Steer clear.

Siberian rhubarb

Siberian rhubarb is traditionally used as a laxative with some evidence that one of the chemicals in the rhubarb might affect oestrogen receptors.

We have one small short-term study that did indeed show its use yielded less menopausal symptoms, but NAMS says we need more studies before we can feel confident about its efficacy and safety.

It comes with a few warnings. Rhubarb leaves contain oxalic acid, which can cause tummy pain, burning of the mouth and throat, diarrhoea, nausea and vomiting. So this is another three Gwyneths.

Dong quai

This herb is commonly used as part of traditional Chinese medicine for the treatment of women's conditions generally. There has been a single clinical trial, which found no benefit from using dong quai for hot flushes. Women on Warfarin (a blood thinner) can't use dong quai. NAMS does not recommend the use of dong quai for relieving hot flushes. Two Gwyneths.

Hypericum (St John's wort)

More often used for anxiety and depression than hot flushes, this herb has been trialled for menopause symptoms but hot flushes have never been specifically singled out in these studies. However, the results so far have been pretty good. In combination with other herbs, and on its own, a meta-analysis of the various studies found that hypericum is 'significantly superior to placebo'. I'd give this a shot *if* you are also getting symptoms of anxiety or depression (see Chapter 5, Somebody burnt down my happy place) *and* your doctor or pharmacist has checked it won't interfere with anything else you're taking. Zero Gwyneths if your moods are suffering on your menopause journey. But do check with your pharmacist or GP. This can't be taken with most standard antidepressant medications.

Vitamin E

Vitamin E was first considered a possible treatment for hot flushes back in the 1940s, but it wasn't until 1998 when the first randomised, cross-over, clinical trial took place. This trial saw 120 women take vitamin E (800 IU daily) for four weeks, then four weeks of placebo or vice versa. It turned out that vitamin E *did* work for hot flushes . . . kind of. It reduced the flushes by *one hot flush* per day. But the women in the study didn't prefer it to the placebo. It's linked to a higher risk of heart failure in other studies; don't bother. Three Gwyneths.

Any other treatments out there?

Magnet therapy

So the idea of magnets being able to alter brain waves and change symptoms isn't new. It has been used successfully for depression and even possibly for migraines. So it shouldn't be surprising that someone invented a magnet for hot flushes, too. These tend to be clipped on to your underwear and you just wear them every day until your symptoms go away. Studies, albeit small, show they don't work. But, unless you have a pacemaker (in which case, avoid them like the plague), they don't have any side effects and I have no problem with a placebo. As they're a one-off purchase, and they claim to last indefinitely, it's not the biggest waste of money out there. So if you're using one and finding it helpful, feel free to continue! One Gwyneth.

Homeopathy

Homeopathy was invented in the 1700s by Samuel Christian Hahnemann, a German physician. Homeopathy's first 'law' is *similia similibus curentur*, or 'let likes be cured by likes'. In other words, microdosing with the agent that gives you the problem will cure you. The 'law of infinitesimal doses' decrees that when agents are diluted in either water or alcohol, they actually increase in therapeutic potency. Today, serial dilutions of 1:100 repeated 6 or 30 times are commonly used. That means there's basically close to none of the original agent left in a homeopathic medicine. Between each dilution the substance is violently shaken, which is thought to be necessary to activate the properties of the drug.

Everything about homeopathy runs counter to science. There is no scientific evidence or even reasonable theory to explain it. The 'law' of infinitesimal doses also runs contrary to everything we know about chemistry, pharmacology and thermodynamics. So, will you be surprised to find that there is no evidence that homeopathy works for hot flushes of menopause? I'm giving a special dispensation though — four Gwyneths from me.

Acupuncture

There is a bit of evidence that acupuncture helps menopausal symptoms. The problem is the positive studies are pretty rubbish. A meta-analysis of six randomised sham-controlled trials (i.e., decent quality studies) concluded that there were no benefits of acupuncture over placebo for hot flushes. But it is good for people due to a decent placebo effect. One Gwyneth.

New horizons

So I mentioned neurokinin B (NKB) and its possible role in hot flushes. We now have a medication targeting NKB. In early studies, menopausal women reported a significant reduction in the number of hot flushes, an 82 per cent decrease in lost sleep and a 77 per cent reduction in lost concentration. Stay tuned! I'll give it a true Gwyneth rating when there are more studies and people start using it.

Do hot flushes say anything about my general health?

More than just a terrible inconvenience, we think having hot flushes puts you at higher risk of heart disease.

A prospective forward-looking study of 11,725 women who enrolled in a trial and were then followed for 14 years found that women who had frequent hot flushes or night sweats had twice the rate of coronary heart disease as women who had no hot flushes. Hot flushes have also been associated with certain cardiovascular risk factors. For example, women with hot flushes seem to have higher levels of LDL (bad) cholesterol, triglycerides and blood inflammatory markers. Plus they are more likely to have diabetes, insulin resistance and high blood pressure. As yet we don't know what lies behind this link.

So if you have been particularly troubled by hot flushes, go to your GP for a blood-pressure check, a cholesterol test and make sure your BMI is at a healthy level — independent of what you do about your hot flushes.

Dr Nicholas Panay says menopause is a good opportunity to check in with a health-care professional anyway and check up on your general health.

From having standard checks such as bowel-cancer screening, mammogram and cervical screening to blood pressure, blood glucose and cholesterol checks, it's a good idea whether you have hot flushes or not.

HOT FLUSHES
THE BOTTOM LINE

Hot flushes can be mildly inconvenient through to unbearable.

HRT is the best way to combat them — hands down.

Not everyone can take HRT and there are other options available, including many prescription medicines.

Herbal remedies might be worth a shot, but none have the same evidence as HRT.

There's a high placebo effect in studies of complementary and alternative therapies for hot flushes. (But who cares? If it works for you, go for it!)

Some complementary remedies have dangerous side effects — tread carefully.

CHAPTER 4

WHAT THE HELL HAPPENED TO MY VAGINA?

You think you've seen my passion already? *This*, girls, is the big issue for me.

If you are lucky enough to roll into your fifties with a rocking great sex life, intact libido, A-grade bladder, strong orgasms and a sweet-smelling, sexy vagina, then good luck to you. You can skip this chapter. For the rest of us, the vagina is often the part of the body that gives us the most consternation.

Studies have found that 45–63 per cent of postmenopausal women report vulvovaginal symptoms. That number climbs to 80 per cent for women aged 65 years and older. And, in my experience, they are *never* talked about. Not between women friends, not mother to daughter and not even to a doctor. (Not even to *me*, and I *love* talking menopause!) As a result, only 7 per cent of women get any treatment, which completely sucks.

For those not familiar, we're talking vaginal and vulvar dryness, burning and irritation, sexual symptoms such as lack of lubrication, vaginal discomfort or pain, and 'impaired function' such as impaired orgasms, arousal and desire. Plus there are urinary symptoms such as needing to pee all the time (urgency) and recurrent urinary tract infections. Together these symptoms make up the tantalisingly named 'Genitourinary Syndrome of Menopause (GSM)'.

You might develop reduced elasticity of the vagina, a higher vaginal pH (more about that in a moment), changes in vaginal bugs or flora, less lubrication and more susceptibility to physical irritation and trauma. I want to stress that this doesn't happen to everyone. I do lots of cervical screening (the old pap tests) on women who've been through menopause and many have no issues in that department. But I feel very passionate about helping those women who have all or some of the symptoms of GSM to gain better access to treatment.

So settle down for a chat about undies that smell like a pub urinal, the multiple excuses for avoiding sex, the embarrassment of bumping into a friend while you're shopping for vaginal lubricants, and the melancholy of watching your love temple morph into a greyer, saggier version of its younger self. Before you head off to drown your sorrows to dismiss this awful image, the news is pretty good: there are excellent treatments.

And you should seriously treat these symptoms. Unlike hot flushes, which will usually get better, GSM is permanent and tends to get worse over time. The later you start treatment, the less helpful the treatments are. So, my sisters, I strongly urge against grinning and bearing it. Get it sorted, ASAP.

I thought it was just me?

Oestrogen receptors are everywhere in the body. They're abundant in not only the vagina and vulva, but also the muscles of the pelvic floor, urethra and bladder. At a cellular level, as oestrogen disappears, the amount of connective tissue (the kind of scaffolding that holds together your lady bits, such as collagen, hyaluronic acid and elastin) drops. This has some pretty intense implications for your urogenital area.

Sex problems in women are common and they're not confined to menopause. The Prevalence of Female Sexual Problems Associated with Distress and Determinants of Treatment Seeking (PRESIDE) study questioned more than 31,000 American women aged between 18 and 102 years about their sexual experiences, habits and any problems. The PRESIDE study found that over 44 per cent of women had a sexual problem. And 12 per cent of women reported having a distressing sexual problem. All of the sexual problems were worse around and after menopause — and then just kept getting worse with age.

I was actually surprised by this. In my practice I'd say that only 44 per cent of women *don't* have a sexual problem!

The loss of oestrogen after menopause causes all of the problems we see women complaining of at this stage of life. Women often avoid sex because of these problems and that can take a heavy toll on their relationships.

Vaginal dryness is a problem in itself. Culturally, women and men both seem to enjoy sex when the vagina is 'wetter'; women seem to be able to orgasm better with a 'wetter' vagina, and painful sex is more likely to occur with a dry vagina. So, with the lack of oestrogen stopping the vagina from producing its own natural lubricant, the entire thing can become fraught.

This is all compounded by the fact that few couples talk about what is happening and lots of men take it very personally. But the menopausal, aging vagina does not have to ruin a sexual relationship. Should you choose to treat it, there are many options out there.

What happens to my body during sex?

I think that, as a woman, you should know what happens from that first sexy thought all the way through to your orgasm. It's sciency, nerdy and incredibly unsexy, but it will give you an appreciation of how complex a system it is, and why it's so easy for things to go wrong.

Sexual arousal starts in the brain. Response to a stimulus (a photo of a shirtless George Clooney — am I showing my age?) triggers your hypothalamus, limbic system and hippocampus in your brain to start to transmit signals through both the parasympathetic and sympathetic nervous systems.

In response to this nervous stimulation, a cascade of chemicals is released from the nerves of the vagina, clitoris and vulva. Some magic happens that we still poorly understand, which results in the blood vessels supplying the clitoris, vagina and labia becoming engorged with blood. Glands in the uterus and the vagina (Bartholin's glands), as well as the vaginal cells themselves, start to secrete lubricating fluids. The muscle walls of the vagina relax and the uterus sits higher in the pelvis — so the entire vagina both lengthens and widens to accommodate the enlarged penis heading its way. Meanwhile, stimulation of the clitoris also makes both its length and width increase as it becomes engorged with blood.

Ultimately, with enough stimulation (which doesn't necessarily have to be genital), you get your reward with major involuntary spasms of various muscle groups in the vagina and around the anus, as well as a spike in heart rate and blood pressure. There's also increased activity in areas of the brain including the hypothalamus, midbrain, hippocampus and cerebellum. Hello orgasm!

During an orgasm, your brain produces a large amount of oxytocin, which is responsible for the contractions of your uterus and also makes you feel closer to your partner and gives you that warm, stress-free, calm, happy feeling. Just before and just after sex, orgasm or not, your testosterone levels rise, although why, we're not quite sure. But you can imagine that a lack of testosterone would play some role in disrupting your sexual function.

How do I fix my sex life?

The first thing to say here is that you don't necessarily need to do anything. If by avoiding sex, you don't feel like you're missing anything, and you're quite happy letting that part of your life sit quietly, please don't worry. That is super common. Many of my patients are not in a sexual relationship and don't need a well-lubricated vagina. They often put a smile on my face by coming in four or five years later to tell me they've met someone and might need that help after all! Some of my patients' partners have medical problems that prevent them getting erections or being able to have any sort of sex at all. Some women are relieved to see it go, some are devastated, and then there's everything in between. I simply want to give you options should you wish to get your sex life back.

Talk to your partner, please. If women aren't talking to their doctors about vaginal symptoms, they certainly don't seem to be talking to their husbands or partners. Let me tell you what I see, and you tell me if this sounds familiar . . . Slowly but surely, some time around menopause, sex starts to change. You can't get as wet as you used to. At times it feels as if you're making love to a sandpaper-covered extra-large dildo that leaves your vagina feeling raw and torn inside. With the pain it is harder to orgasm. You don't know whether to yell 'Stop!' or just hope he gets it over and done with as quickly as possible. Sex is certainly not something you look forward to. So you make excuses. You delay going to bed, or try to race to bed and pretend to be asleep before he gets there. Because just the thought of having sex makes you really anxious. He knows there's something wrong but he's just not sure what's going on. Nobody talks about it. Even without the pain, your libido has often just completely vanished. He asks for sex a couple of times, gets rebuffed and gets annoyed, or aggressive: 'What's wrong with you?' It's hard to be attracted to someone when the thought of sex is just so terrifying.

Even women in same-sex relationships can experience this, especially when there is a significant age gap between you. This problem freezes couples apart. It doesn't cause World War III, just a slow and growing chasm between you.

If you don't explain what is happening, it can become a huge rift in your relationship. Please swallow your pride and just talk honestly to him (or her). 'It's not you, it's just me,' might be a cliché but your partner really needs to hear this and understand. It's medical; it's biological; it's not about your partner's lack of sex appeal! But let the ground between you freeze over and it will cause even bigger issues. Ask him to come with you to the GP to get help. Sex is a two-person issue. He can hear from your doctor what is going on and join your attempts to fix it.

So, what treatments are available and work best?

A British study published in *Maturitas* in April 2019 found that when it comes to GSM, the most common treatment was non-hormonal therapy applied vaginally (31.8 per cent), followed by hormonal therapy applied vaginally (11.6 per cent) and systemic hormonal therapy (4.7 per cent). You need to keep reading to understand my sadness at these statistics.

Why are so few women using what works?

We know how much these symptoms affect them and how common they are. Is it that they're too scared? Or is it, as I suspect, that their doctors aren't giving my sisters the option of the most effective treatments for this condition?

Dr Nicholas Panay, General Secretary of the International Menopause Society (IMS), is the author of the 2019 *Maturitas* study. In his experience, there are barriers to women seeking any treatment at all for GSM. 'Women perceive vaginal dryness as inevitable,' he told me. He added that they're too embarrassed to bring it up with their health-care professional. They don't want to delve into their relationship issues, especially with a stranger. But, what he found fascinating is that, despite all of that, if their health-care professional brings it up, more than 80 per cent of women are actually happy to have a chat about it. So doctors need to do better.

I'm listing the treatments below, starting with the big guns because hormone treatment works for GSM. *It just does*. The issue honestly is starting it early enough and continuing it long enough. 'If therapy is delayed for too long, vulvovaginal atrophy changes can become less reversible or irreversible, regardless of the type of therapy used,' according to Dr Panay. Having said that, it's never too late to at least give it a shot.

Vaginal oestrogen

Creams and tablets (and the 90-day rings, which are hardly used) containing low-dose oestrogen can be inserted directly into the vagina or (in the case of the cream) rubbed directly onto the vulva. The huge advantage of vaginal oestrogen is that, if GSM symptoms are the main source of bother, you can deal with them very effectively with minimal absorption into the rest of the body. This means that the oestrogen doesn't need to be counteracted with progesterone.

Vaginal oestrogens are used every night for two to three weeks to get started, then twice a week (sometimes three times) for as long as having a good functioning vagina is important to you. It does take a few weeks to get the full benefits in your vulva and vagina, but in my experience it can transform the lives of patients. Most importantly, the evidence suggests that vaginal oestrogen can be continued for as long as needed. That might be forever.

Very little is absorbed. In fact, one year on vaginal oestrogen gives you the same amount of additional oestrogen in your body as *one day* on HRT. Despite this, the package insert has dire warnings about breast cancer, endometrial cancer and blood-clot risks, for Pete's sake! As Dr Panay said, 'The disclaimers are absolutely ridiculous!' Please don't let them put you off. Fixing this is important for your wellbeing.

Full HRT

It won't surprise you to know that hot flushes around menopause correlate with low libido and low enjoyment of sex. While many of my patients tell me going on HRT is life-changing for their sex life, others report that their HRT is not enough to fix their GSM. In fact, studies show that between 10 and 25 per cent of women taking HRT still have symptoms of GSM, even when their flushes are totally sorted. In that case, adding vaginal oestrogen on top of the HRT usually fixes it.

Tibolone

We met the medication Tibolone as a treatment for hot flushes in Chapter 3. It gets broken into a chemical that mimics some of the effects of oestrogen but not others. It's great for bones, great for hot flushes but, most importantly when it comes to your sex life, it is also partially broken down into testosterone. While that's not the full story, experts analysing the studies say that Tibolone can benefit libido — so it's at least worth considering. You might still need a tiny bit of vaginal oestrogen as a top-up.

Testosterone

This is a bit of a passion of mine. Lack of access to testosterone (either because pharmaceutical companies don't make it for women or because the products available aren't approved by government bodies, for archaic historical reasons) is a reason many patients are driven to clinics selling 'bio-identical hormones'. So many women passionately want a sex life. They don't need to be swinging from the chandeliers and it doesn't need to be every night. But they don't want the sense of dread that comes from the tap on the shoulder heralding pain, discomfort and malaise.

Here's how I approach sexual problems in menopause: I'm assuming first that the relationship is good and doesn't need fixing. So first I get a diagnosis. Is it just low desire or are there issues with vaginal dryness and atrophy, too? In most cases there are, so I fix GSM first. I don't care how high your libido is, if sex feels like sandpaper being rammed into your vagina, your sex life won't get any better! If we fix that and you still have no desire and/or can't enjoy orgasms the way you could, I would consider testosterone cream.

Taking testosterone isn't a new concept. We know that low testosterone levels in the blood of women after menopause correlate with low libido. It is over 60 years since testosterone therapy was first tried for postmenopausal women with sexual problems. Its role is to fix libido in menopausal women who fit the criteria for 'Hypoactive Sexual Desire Disorder'. In many women, it is the only thing that works. Over the years, different doses and regimens have been tried, in combination with oestrogen/progesterone or on its own. And most (but not all) studies suggest that testosterone improves sexual dysfunction in postmenopausal women, regardless of whether it comes as a skin cream or patches, or as a tablet. It does this without any effect on vaginal dryness.

In the UK and Australia it comes as a cream that you rub on your upper thighs or belly every day. You start by rubbing in 0.5ml and increase that as required with the help of your doctor to a maximum of 1.5ml a day. We monitor your blood testosterone levels to make sure you're on the right dose, especially initially.

Many doctors have been cautious. Certainly in theory, pumping more testosterone into your body could be expected to cause heart disease, high cholesterol, unwanted hair growth, acne and vaginal bleeding. Well, it can: but it's not as common as you'd think and it tends to be mild. We are using very tiny doses — much lower than the doses used by men who have low testosterone. In the case of heart disease, it's not absolutely clear that testosterone does increase the risk at all. And, in case you've heard rumours, well-managed testosterone therapy in women doesn't produce acne, a hoarse voice, aggression or a beard! Having said that, most of the studies are short (around 52 weeks maximum) so we can't say there's no risk, just that the risks don't show up in the first year.

Who can have it? Well, we do need blood tests first. I test your testosterone and SHBG (sex hormone-binding globulin) levels as well as your cholesterol. Because, according to the IMS, while there is no cut-off level of testosterone or any other androgen that will identify women most likely to respond to testosterone, treatment with testosterone is less likely to be effective in women with a SHBG level above the normal range. The IMS recommendation is that a testosterone level is checked three weeks after starting therapy and then routinely every six months, with dose adjustment if the levels become higher than the top of the normal range for women.

The maximum benefit isn't seen for four to six weeks, and if you're not getting any benefit after six months, we'd stop the treatment and try something different. When I prescribe testosterone for a patient, I monitor her closely for cholesterol, blood pressure and weight to make sure she is carefully managing the risk factors for heart disease (just in case there is a risk that has not yet been detected by the studies to date).

I really hope that for women with low desire, they get better access to testosterone formulations sooner rather than later. This will take more progressive government legislation and better training of doctors. I spoke to Michael Buckley, who manufactures the testosterone cream that most doctors with a special interest in menopause prescribe in Australia and the UK. He advised me that doctors (that includes GPs and specialists) who belong to their countries' Menopause Societies are familiar with prescribing testosterone cream. So he suggests seeking out a doctor who will be on board with your wishes by using the 'find a doctor' service on your country's Menopause Society website. Good advice indeed.

You can also get testosterone through the compounded testosterone 'pellet' inserted by doctors who prescribe bio-identical hormones; it's just harder to adjust the dose. I've already told you my thoughts on getting HRT through bio-identical hormones. A lot of these prescribers tend to also separately prescribe you some DHEA, which they have compounded.

This isn't a grey area: the IMS's 2018 *Sexual Wellbeing After Menopause* white paper *clearly stated* that systematic reviews of the clinical trials of DHEA for women have shown no significant effect on sexual function, and they have warned women off using it at all, for any sexual problem. Ditto the 'love hormone', oxytocin, which is prescribed for sexual problems. Indeed, oxytocin appears to improve 'emotional responsiveness' (responding in a more emotionally appropriate way to your partner) in some small studies, but this hasn't translated well into the sexual space. In fact, oxytocin has been found to be useless in studies for the treatment of sexual dysfunction in women.

Dr Fiona Jane is a specialist women's health GP at Jean Hailes for Women's Health in Melbourne. She points out that testosterone is not a panacea: 'It is important that women understand that testosterone is not going to make a poor relationship better and is effective in about 50 per cent of cases.'

Candy's story

I had firsthand experience of this as a GP. I had been seeing Candy as a patient for about 10 years. She'd been in a monogamous relationship with a guy for maybe 15 years and had been on antidepressants on and off since her first marriage broke down almost 30 years ago. And she had had a hysterectomy before I met her. So, picking the exact time of menopause was a bit tricky in that situation. But a lot happened at once. She started with hot flushes at about age 54, and her libido took a serious nosedive. It was impacting on her relationship and she was in a terrible way when she came to see me.

Her priorities were fixing her flushing and rebooting her libido. They were equally important to her. We went through her options and decided that, even though she didn't need progesterone to counter oestrogen (having no uterus, post-hysterectomy), we could tick both boxes using Tibolone.

The problem for Candy was massive, debilitating depression. Tibolone can, and in Candy's case did, throw depression into hyperdrive. Within four weeks Candy was practically not functioning. Her depression had got so bad she couldn't sleep; she couldn't cope with household practicalities and everyday duties. We had to get her off Tibolone ASAP.

Plan B worked a treat. We opted for an oestrogen patch and, after a blood test, testosterone cream. Within four days of stopping the Tibolone, Candy said she felt a weight lifting off her shoulders. She's back in therapy, back at work and just coping generally so much better. The testosterone took a little longer (around six weeks) to kick in. We needed a baseline testosterone level, and we're monitoring her testosterone, cholesterol and blood pressure. All good so far. And she is actually back to enjoying sex again.

Rachel's story

Rachel is 57. She went through menopause at age 52 and only had a few very manageable hot flushes, and her mood was absolutely fine. She's really fit, being a tennis coach, and has a very attractive husband. They travel and have a great life. But when I saw her for a cervical screening test (the one we used to call a pap test), I noticed her vagina was very dry and so I asked her how she was doing in the bedroom department.

She wasn't, she admitted. Over the past few years she had found sex increasingly uncomfortable and her libido had gone south shortly thereafter. She and her husband had started having sex less and less often and now neither of them mentioned it. She missed her libido but thought this was just an inevitable part of getting old. At 57? Hell no!

First stop, a vaginal moisturiser every third day and a vaginal oestrogen cream. I saw her three months later and she was finding sex bearable, but she still had no libido. A blood test confirmed she was suitable for testosterone cream. I remember her starting it just before they were off on a holiday. I warned her it takes a while to be effective. By the time she came back for her follow-up blood test only a matter of weeks later, she was bursting with excitement. I've never needed to increase Rachel's dose. She's got her sex life back and this has led to all sorts of improvements in other areas of her relationship. This won't happen to everyone but it happens to a lot of women. Chat to your GP if you think this could be a winner for you.

Hormone therapy is definitely not for me . . . what else could I do to improve my sex life?

Get enough sleep

This is easy low-hanging fruit. In my practice I see a lot of women who are just so ridiculously busy they don't have enough hours in the day, and sleep deprivation is almost the norm. I'm guilty of this, too. While we feel exhausted and are aware of the general brain fug, we often don't put two and two together and associate our rapidly declining sex life with our lack of zzzzzz.

According to the International Society for Sexual Medicine, research shows that women with partners have a higher libido the day after a good night's sleep than after a bad night. And sleeping longer leads to more arousal and a higher chance of actually having sex the next day. How much sleep? A study of postmenopausal women found that women who sleep less than seven hours each night are less likely to say they feel sexually satisfied.

Sleep deprivation has a few effects on your sex life. Firstly, your hottest bedroom fantasy might involve closed curtains, a pillow and being left alone. For an exhausted woman, sleep trumps sex in any position. In a contest between sleep and the 10 or 20 minutes required to achieve orgasm, the orgasm doesn't stand a chance.

Plus sleep deprivation wreaks havoc with relationships. You are more likely to snap at your partner, be critical, annoyed and frustrated, and less likely to notice how cute he looks in that new shirt. (See page 90 for some tips on fixing the relationship.) So get a good night's sleep ASAP. And then get another, and another, and another . . .

Lubricants and moisturisers

While we're waiting for vaginal oestrogen to kick in, if that's the direction you've chosen, or while we're waiting for your relationship to light up, lubricants and moisturisers can right a lot of short-term wrongs.

Lubricants certainly make sex less uncomfortable and take the pressure off before the act so you don't have to worry about whether or not it will hurt. There are a ton of vaginal lubricants on the market. Sadly, although the ingredients are listed on the box, they read as scientific gobbledy gook.

Professor Gayle Fischer is a clinical and academic dermatologist with an interest in gynaecological dermatology. She has published numerous articles about the vulva and vagina, and is a member of the International Society for the Study of Vulvar Disease. Her advice on lubricants is that you don't necessarily need a specifically formulated product. A really small amount of a pure vegetable oil or olive oil contains no irritating chemicals, preservatives or perfumes. Her favourite is coconut oil. It rinses off pretty easily in water and doesn't increase the risk of vaginal infection. Petroleum jelly (such as Vaseline) is also extremely unlikely to cause irritation. She advises women to steer clear of any water-based products such as K-Y Jelly and other branded lubricants. She explains that many contain alcohol and an antiseptic called chlorhexidine that can actually dry out the vagina. Exactly what the doctor didn't order!

I'd avoid parabens, glycerol, glycerine and propylene glycol (which can cause vaginal irritation). I'd also be careful *not* to use products that can destroy condoms if you're not yet through menopause and that's your contraception of choice. Unfortunately, all of the oils I mentioned in the previous paragraph fall into this category and can make your condoms totally unreliable. So, armed with all this advice, head online and search for lubricants without those ingredients. They are out there!

The time taken to the 'end of the road' is important! Too inexplicit? Let me be more blunt . . . If your partner ejaculates fairly quickly, then often a lubricant is all you need. But if your partner lasts a long time before ejaculation, the lubricant is often *initially* awesome and then . . . it stops being so awesome. So you'll need something else.

Moisturisers rehydrate the vulvar and vaginal tissues, and lower the pH. They can be used every day, or even just every third day, to increase the health of the vagina. There are moisturisers you can insert into the vagina and moisturisers made specifically for the vulva.

Vaginal moisturisers should ideally be paraben-free, and have an osmolality below the 'WHO ideal recommendation of 380mOsm/kg'. WTF? I have looked through hundreds of websites and can hardly find any products that even *mention* pH or 'osmolality', let alone reveal their numbers. I did find one — a US brand — that addresses all of these issues but I can't name it because the Australian government says that would constitute my advertising a product, and doctors aren't allowed to advertise. The important thing is, it's worth using a moisturiser. One study showed that using a vaginal moisturiser containing hyaluronic acid gel every three days improves vaginal dryness, and was comparable to topical oestrogen therapy.

When it comes to the vulva, Professor Fischer warns women to avoid moisturisers containing preservatives, which can make the area even more sensitive. 'Use an emulsifying ointment on the vulva,' she advises. In this case, an emulsifying ointment means a mixture of paraffin oils used to moisturise very dry skin. It is greasy and so it leaves a layer of oil on the vulval skin that traps water in the skin and hydrates it.

Get some exercise

This is one of the best interventions for sexual problems; there are studies that have actually looked at this. Without a doubt, people who regularly work out have more sex, and enjoy sex more. It could be that fitness allows you to go another couple of rounds, or just better body image in general. Feeling flabby and unattractive won't put too many of us in the mood for sex. Plus, we know regular exercise has a powerful effect on mood and, in turn, low mood and low sexual function are regular bedfellows. (Excuse the dad joke.)

Whatever the link, the jury is in . . . Do more exercise and not only will you boost your mood, lose weight, prevent and manage chronic diseases and sleep better, but we'll throw in a better sex life for free.

Get your hot flushes sorted

Having hot flushes, especially at night, not only leaves you exhausted, but also makes sweaty, intense, personal contact very uncomfortable. I am aware that we keep looping back between chapters, but fixing hot flushes, if you have them, is a bit of a theme. As I already mentioned, the more severe the hot flushes, the more uncomfortable sex is, as a general rule.

Get your medical problems sorted

Medical problems can definitely affect your libido. Whether you have a sore hip from arthritis, making sex an adventure in agony, or you're so tired from breathlessness that anything more than sitting still leaves you exhausted, you need to sort out your unmanaged diseases. See your GP and discuss the impact of these conditions on your sex life to see whether their management can be improved.

If you don't have any obvious medical problems, you should still get checked for low iron and underactive thyroid. Both of these are easy to diagnose and fix (either with iron-replacement therapy or thyroid-replacement therapy) and if that's all that stands between you and a killer sex life, then you're laughing!

Medication review

If you take medication for medical problems, head to your GP or pharmacist for a medication review. So many really common medications can cause sexual problems. For example, all sorts of blood-pressure medicines, such as Clonidine, Lisinopril and Metoprolol, can interfere with both your libido and your ability to reach orgasm. Strong painkillers are real libido killers as well. Ditto lots of the sleeping or anti-anxiety pills, such as Diazepam, Alprazolam and Lorazepam. (I *hate* all of these because they are so addictive and can leave you drowsy and accident prone the next day, so I hope you're not taking them!) Many antidepressants are libido killers, as is the pill if you haven't hit full-blown menopause yet. In almost every case, there is an alternative that won't destroy your sex life, but *you* have to raise the issue with your health-care professional — if they don't know it's bothering you, they're unlikely to bring up the option of switching medications.

Listen out for new drugs coming up

In the US and Europe, preparations are available to improve many of the symptoms of GSM that affect the vagina, but at this time, they're not available in Australia. For example, Ospemifeme is a selective estrogen receptor modulator (SERM) that works specifically to increase the health of the vagina. Another one we can't get in Australia yet is a daily-dose vaginal gel of DHEA (Prasterone) that converts to oestrogen and testosterone in the vagina. Women who have access love these, and I can't wait until we get them here.

Strengthen your pelvic floor muscles

These are the bane of pregnant women, who are all constantly reminded to do pelvic floor (or Kegel) exercises. Well, it turns out that doing so will not only prevent you from having a little overflow accident every time you cough or run for the bus, but pelvic floor exercises can also make sex more enjoyable, increase the intensity of your orgasms and increase your libido. They do this by increasing the strength and also your awareness of the muscles involved in pleasurable sexual sensations, and that can help some women achieve orgasm. They also reduce vaginal or pelvic pain during sex, probably by ensuring the muscles relax during sex. And improving some forms of urinary incontinence makes you less self-conscious in the bedroom. To perform these exercises, tighten your pelvic muscles as if you're stopping a stream of urine. Hold for a count of two to three seconds, relax and repeat. The North American Menopause Society (NAMS) recommends you do these exercises in five sets of 10 repetitions per day.

NAMS also recommends yoga to improve your sex life! Yoga is not only relaxing, but it also focuses your attention on sensation and strengthens pelvic muscles — many yoga poses exercise these muscles. Yoga also improves your own self-image and has all the usual benefits of exercise. In one US study of women of all ages undergoing a 12-week yoga program, three out of four women reported improvements in desire, arousal, lubrication, orgasm, satisfaction and pain reduction. The biggest improvements were in women aged 45 or older.

Get some counselling

Stress and relationship issues can wreak havoc on your libido, so getting them sorted can make a huge difference to your sex life. Sexual counselling is a curious area that tends to be pretty poorly regulated. I can't tell you how to find a good sex therapist, but, in my experience, if a couple is keen on exploring tantra and the use of sex toys with a sex therapist, they're usually doing pretty well and probably don't need one!

The sort of therapy I'm talking about is, of course, couples counselling — with someone who is well equipped to discuss the intricacies of your physical relationship as well. Someone who can integrate the physical, the spiritual and the emotional aspects of your love life.

Hopefully your GP will be able to make a recommendation but if not, call around — some psychologists and counsellors are more comfortable than others and they should be pretty up-front if you make an inquiry.

Stress control

Stress is cyanide for your libido. When your head is consumed with worries and anxiety, it can be impossible to be able to think about sex or orgasms. If I had a simple, straightforward, stress-nuking formula, I promise I would give it to you. I think it's important to acknowledge the role that stress plays in taking out your libido and your ability to really get into sex the way you'd like to.

If you are going through a short-term stressful period, such as uncertainty about your role at work or a serious illness in a family member or friend, make the link and then take the pressure off yourself. Hopefully the situation will settle down and your sexual appetite and enjoyment will return to normal with it.

If you are facing protracted stress from financial woes, serious relationship breakdown or illness, then that's a different story. Sure, your sex life could fall apart, but so might your physical and mental health and your sleep. You're at risk of drug and alcohol issues and poor performance at work. There are so many reasons to tackle this issue. And, to be honest, fixing your sex life might be a relatively minor one.

The problem I find with many of my patients is they don't necessarily recognise it. They're so mired in the morass of stress that they can't see the effect it's having on them. If they could take a step back — as I do as their GP, being an impartial third party looking at the situation — they would definitely want to do whatever it takes to feel better.

Daniel, my husband, always says: 'Life's not just about getting a good hand, but about playing a bad hand well.' It is about being able to manage the situation you're in better, so that stressful events don't take such a massive toll on you. Whether you choose prayer and church, the comfort of close friends, rigorous exercise or meditation is up to you. And most people need to try a few different things to find the one that works. If nothing works, get yourself some help. Start with your GP to get referred to a great counsellor or psychologist.

What about vaginal discharge?

Acid in the vagina is your friend. Before menopause, the overwhelming majority of the bugs or 'microbes' in the vagina are lactobacilli. Lactobacillus is an awesome bug: its superpowers come from the fact that it ferments carbohydrates to lactic acid. That gives the vagina a low (or acidic) pH. The normal vagina has a pH of 3.8. This acid environment is toxic to many nastier microbes. When levels of lactobacilli drop, the pH becomes more alkaline, so the risk of infection rises. In fact, increasing the pH of the vagina to anywhere over 4.5 dramatically increases the odds of an infection from bugs such as *Gardnerella vaginalis* (the non-sexually transmitted, fishy-smelling bacteria that many women worry about), *Chlamydia trachomatis* (a sexually transmitted infection), *Candida albicans* (thrush) and *E. coli* and other bacteria that cause urinary tract infections.

As you start heading towards menopause, the bugs in the vagina begin to change and the proportion of lactobacillus bacteria starts to drop. They make up 83 per cent of the microbiota in premenopausal women, 83 per cent in perimenopausal women and 54 per cent in postmenopausal women.

The result?

Some women end up getting bacterial vaginosis — a non-sexually transmitted infection that generally causes a smelly vaginal discharge, clear to grey in colour. Around 50 per cent of women with it get no symptoms. If you do get symptoms, they are most likely going to be related to the odour and maybe an itch. We rarely see burning and stinging per se, but given this goes with a postmenopausal vagina anyway, the two might accidentally coincide.

While it isn't a sexually transmitted infection (STI), it *does* increase your risk of picking up an STI that you encounter. So, there's extra impetus to treat it if you're not in a monogamous relationship. Here are some pointers about how to deal with it and look after your vagina in general.

Douching

Hand on heart, before I became a GP I'd never heard of this. So, excuse me if I take a moment to explain it. Vaginal douching is the process of 'intra-vaginal cleansing' with a liquid solution. People add vinegar, bleach, iodine, yoghurt, bicarbonate of soda and anything else they can think of into the douching water. Women douche to 'clean out' their vagina.

The problem with it is that the forceful insertion of water pushes bacteria up further into the vagina and uterus, where they shouldn't be. And at the same time it removes your own healthy bacteria. Indeed, the scientific studies of douching link it to all sorts of horrific medical problems, including pelvic inflammatory disease, bacterial vaginosis, cervical cancer, pregnancy problems, HIV transmission and other sexually transmitted diseases, recurrent thrush and infertility. *Just don't do it!*

Soap, bubble bath and shower gels

Soap is *so bad* for a vagina of any age, but especially around menopause. It disrupts the chemistry of the vagina and dries out and irritates the vulvar skin (making you itch). If you insist on using anything other than plain water, I have two pieces of advice: no soap (only use a mild soap-free cleanser); and stick to skin that has (or once had) hair on it. Never on pink bits! For pink (totally hairless) bits, as an alternative to water, you can use a simple perfume-free moisturiser like Sorbelene as you would a soap, and then rinse with water. No matter what you do, only wash once a day — your vulva needs no more than that.

Perfume

Don't laugh. Lots of women are horrified by their own smell and use 'body sprays' and perfumes directly onto the vulva. You might have got away with that in your twenties, when the vulval skin is robust, but at menopause the alcohol in perfume and the preservatives will make any vulval dermatitis and water loss from the skin worse.

Wipes

Scented or otherwise, wipes (even baby wipes) are incredibly bad for the environment and often contain preservatives that can make vulval dermatitis worse.

Rough drying

If your skin is inflamed, rubbing it dry with a towel is going to inflame it even more. Pat dry gently or even blow-dry your vulva with a hair dryer on a cool setting.

Yoghurt up the fanny?

Lots of my patients try putting yoghurt into their vagina. There's just no evidence for it, and it is messy and in theory could put all the wrong bugs into the fanny. Not recommended.

Some antibiotics directly into the vagina will sort the issue out very quickly. You do need a script from your doctor, which does make for an embarrassing conversation if you don't have a doc you feel completely comfortable with. My advice? Get the consultation over and done with and embark on a journey to find your dream GP. This is a time of your life where that relationship is critical.

What is causing my itchy fanny?

OK, now this is serious. Women are not big fans of chatting about their itchy fannies. Instead they toddle off to the pharmacy and spend a bucketload on stuff that probably doesn't work and can make the problem worse. Here are some of the reasons it could be itchy.

Just menopause itself

At least in theory, itching can be one of the symptoms of menopause itself and represents one of the issues with atrophic vaginitis (reduced vagina and vulvar tissues). We don't know why some women get an itch rather than pain or urine symptoms. The condition is driven by low oestrogen to the vagina and vulva, and the subsequent atrophy or shrinking of the cells of the vulva.

The fanny is more delicate after menopause. For a start, oestrogen deficiency and just normal aging lower the 'barrier function' of the skin of the vulva, making it more prone to dryness. This dryness, together with the increasing pH (as we just discussed), lowers the immune function of the vulvar skin. This skin also makes less natural lubricating oils, which means it is less able to heal in response to injury.

Besides general steps to reduce itch, it can be treated with oestrogen. Because the lack of oestrogens is the cause of atrophic vaginitis, replacing the oestrogen is the most logical choice of treatment. Plus HRT has proved to be effective in fixing the symptoms. HRT restores your vagina's normal pH levels. It also repairs a healthy blood supply to the vulva and vagina, and increases the number of cells in the vulva and vagina. The oestrogen is usually given locally into the vagina, but if you're on HRT for hot flushes, your vulva and vagina may benefit, too.

Dermatitis

So, the most common cause of an itchy fanny is actually vulvar dermatitis. Symptoms often go beyond itching to extreme itching, rawness, stinging, burning and even pain. Specialist dermatologist Professor Gayle Fischer says this condition is more common in women who have generally sensitive skin and are prone to hay fever, asthma and other 'allergic' conditions.

Any extra irritants can make dermatitis worse. Soap dries the vulva skin out and makes it more alkaline. Ammonia in urine from incontinence chemically irritates the vulva, as can some of the ingredients in the creams women use to try to fix the problem: chemicals such as propylene glycol, parabens and fragrances. Even pads and your underpants can actually physically irritate the vulva.

We treat it by getting rid of any irritants. Your soap, perfume, the undies you're wearing, the pads you're using to protect you from your leaky bladder . . . we'll slather on some petroleum jelly to allow the skin to heal itself. If that doesn't work, we'd use some corticosteroid cream to get rid of the itch. I get really frustrated because when you buy the cream, the leaflet inside the box scares the life out of you and specifically tells you it's not to be used on the genitals. That's not right. Every major gynaecology body recommends steroid preparations for this dermatitis. Given that dermatitis of the vulva can drive you crazy, with anything from an itch to full-on burning, you need the right treatment for this condition.

People are terrified by the word steroid. So, let me put your mind at ease. For dermatitis, you won't be using it forever. It's a short-term anti-inflammatory to settle down a horrible, embarrassing itch.

Lichen sclerosus

So if you're itchy down there, can I ask you to just grab a mirror and have a quick look at your vulva? If you are getting intense itching, especially at night, and there are any pale or even white patches on your vulva, you could be developing lichen sclerosus, a chronic inflammation condition of the vulva.

What does it look like? Well, areas of the vulva affected by lichen sclerosus can look white, even silvery, and be shiny or have a kind of crinkly texture. It can extend from the clitoris down to the anus.

If you do have it, go to a dermatologist or gynaecologist because in 5 per cent of cases it can turn cancerous. That's rare. In all my years of general practice, it has happened to a few women. But still, it's best to get checked out.

Treatment is simple: just corticosteroids on the vulva will help get rid of the itch and control the underlying condition. Plus regular check-ups with your doctor once or twice a year to make sure it's not getting worse. If you do have lichen sclerosus, the steroid treatment usually needs to be forever.

Thrush

I'm going to whiz past this, because it won't usually happen after menopause. That is just because thrush loves plump, healthy, oestrogen-fed cells. However, it does happen in women on HRT or taking vaginal oestrogen. And it does happen in poorly controlled diabetics.

The telltale signs are cheesy white vaginal discharge and swollen, red vulva, often with little paper-cut looking tears in the labia. If in doubt, get it checked out by your doctor. Most postmenopausal women I see with an itchy fanny have already tried thrush cream anyway — and failed — so they're well aware it's not thrush by the time I see them.

General steps for an itchy fanny

1. Don't scratch. It's hard, but scratching sets up an 'itch–scratch' cycle so that the skin can't ever heal and the problem just gets worse.
2. No soap (or shampoo, shower gel, bath salts or bubble bath). I know what you're thinking but I swear you don't need soap down there. Just water. And no 'wipes' or scented toilet paper.
3. Switch to cotton undies, with no panty liners.
4. Try an antihistamine: it often takes the edge off.
5. Be careful of moisturising creams, especially if they contain fragrances. You want an emollient — simple petroleum jelly is a good one — that just creates a barrier but allows your own skin to heal itself.
6. Use icepacks to ease the symptoms.
7. Don't use thrush cream. Unless you're taking HRT or vaginal oestrogen cream, we hardly ever see thrush in postmenopausal women so it's probably not the culprit.

Laser vaginal rejuvenation

Just a quick word on this before we leave your vagina alone. It took the market by storm, promising a 'youthful' and collagenful vagina in a few simple sessions. The various devices on the market use tiny pinpoint laser pulses directly into the vagina. When they first came out, lots of doctors rushed to buy one of the devices, rightly seeing a great market for them. Experts around the world have started to yank the reins on this entire industry, claiming the proof of benefit is minimal and there are lots of potential harms — from scarring your credit card, to scarring and even completely obstructing the vagina itself. Ouch.

Good studies are underway right now, so I'm urging you to hold on to your wallet a bit longer before shelling out for what can only be called an experimental treatment.

Now can we talk about my bladder?

Moving away from your vagina for a moment, let's talk about your pee. Urinary symptoms of GSM tend to not be discussed, which is bizarre when 80 per cent of women in menopause experience some kind of urine issue.

Hitting 50 can feel like you've just turned two again. When you need to go, you *need to go now*. Waiting for an extra few minutes can be catastrophic. And go you do . . . often and through the night. Accidents? Hmm. As for coughing, sneezing, running, jumping (like netball or some aerobic exercise activities), well, they might become high-risk activities. First symptoms of GSM itself include burning or stinging when you wee, constantly feeling like you need to pee (not necessarily from a urinary tract infection or UTI), peeing more frequently at night, urinary incontinence and recurrent UTI.

Urine problems tend to go hand in hand with vaginal problems. In one large observational study of 45- to 60-year-old women, those reporting vaginal dryness were almost twice as likely to report incontinence. It's pretty unpleasant: people with incontinence report significantly lower work productivity and sexual satisfaction, higher rates of major depressive symptoms and less physical activity. And yet, despite this high negative impact, and how common it is, less than a quarter of women ask their doctor about it! Sisters, we need to do better! And I completely understand that we doctors need to make it easier to talk about, too.

So, why have I started wetting myself?

It isn't as straightforward as it sounds and there is much we don't know. Here's what we do know: there are stacks of oestrogen receptors in the bladder wall *and* we know that menopause brings with it a whole heap of changes to the bladder. So we figure the oestrogen does *something* to the bladder; we just don't know exactly what. And it's not just after menopause: 37 per cent of women report a deterioration in symptoms prior to menopause.

Menopause also causes other changes to the urinary organs. For example, the urethra — the pipe that takes urine from the bladder to the vulva (or penis in men) — shortens and its lining becomes thinner. As a direct result, the urethra and the bladder valve can't close as tightly, increasing the risk of incontinence.

To complicate things, getting older also has major impacts on your bladder. For a start, the bladder wall changes. The elastic tissue becomes tough, the bladder can't stretch as well and the bladder muscles weaken. Plus your bladder wall is constantly trying to contract throughout your life — nothing to do with urination. When you're younger, most of these contractions are blocked by nerves from your spinal cord and brain, but the number of sporadic contractions that are not blocked increases with age. These random bladder contractions can give you episodes of urinary incontinence. The bladder also becomes less efficient at fully emptying when you pee, so you get more and more 'residual urine' left over in your bladder as you get older. This creates a higher risk of urinary tract infections.

Bladder leakage is a major issue for women in my practice, even those who have never had children. You start to become aware of urine incontinence, so you get to know every public toilet in your daily life, often taking a pre-emptive pee in toilets you used to think you'd rather die than enter. If this sounds familiar, you're not alone. Sixty per cent of women report incontinence at some point in their lives, so if you don't have it, consider yourself lucky.

There are three major causes of bladder leakage in women: stress, urge and mixed incontinence. Stress incontinence is when putting stress on your bladder, by for example coughing, sneezing or exercising, causes urine leakage. This can start when you're much younger. It is really caused by stretching of the pelvic floor muscles or some minor damage to the nerves of the pelvic floor, most often during childbirth. But is also made worse by obesity, a chronic cough and constipation.

Urge incontinence (also called an 'overactive bladder') is also super common. It involves frequently feeling like you need to pee, and therefore going to the toilet often (including more than once during the night). Data collected in Belgium from women aged 40 years or over visiting their GP revealed that urgency and nocturia (peeing through the night) were the most annoying symptoms for women. Another Finnish study of women found that they rated urge incontinence as more distressing than stress incontinence. Urge incontinence seems to be just a thing that happens with aging and has less to do with oestrogen or a lack thereof. It is also made worse by fizzy drinks, caffeine and constipation.

Most common by far is a bit of both types thrown in together, which we refer to as mixed incontinence.

You might know your bladder isn't working as well as it used to, but knowing what type of incontinence you have will determine the treatment so it is worth putting in the energy to figuring it out. The first step is a fluid and peeing diary. This is often enough to tell the doctor what your problem is. But sometimes we need to go a step further and use tests called urodynamic studies. These assess how well the bladder, sphincters (stoppers or one-way valves) and urethra are storing and releasing urine, as well as your sensations of fullness and urinary urge. There are many different types and every specialist uses their own unique combination of tests. But they might fill your bladder with water using a catheter, and you might need to be filmed doing a pee. (I'm just warning you because some of my patients were shocked by this.)

What can I do about bladder leakage?

Lose some weight

If you are overweight, less pressure on the bladder from excess weight helps all types of incontinence. A systematic review of studies on urge incontinence and metabolic syndrome (a cluster of conditions that includes central or abdominal obesity, cholesterol problems, hypertension, insulin resistance and abnormal sugar levels) found that women with a BMI over 30 are twice as likely to have urge incontinence as women with a BMI less than 24. We think it is about the type of fat you're carrying and the state of inflammation in your body, too.

Manage your constipation

Constipation means more matter in your pelvic area, putting more stress on your pelvic floor and bladder. Given how common constipation is around menopause, it's worth sorting out regardless.

No more fizzy drinks and less caffeine

Both have been linked to urge incontinence. Most pelvic floor special-ists advise *no* fizzy drinks at all and only one caffeinated drink a day. (Horrible, I know!)

Drink earlier in the day

This might sound obvious but stop drinking fluids at least two to three hours before bedtime, with the exception of a sip of fluid to take medica-tions as needed. You still need to aim to drink 2 litres of fluids each day, so drink more in the morning and early afternoon.

Train your bladder

This is best for urge incontinence to ensure your body is responding properly to the cues of bladder fullness. The aim is to retrain your pelvic muscles and your brain to stop feeling and responding to that urgency to pee between actual pees. Here's how you do it:

1. Remain totally still when your urine urgency occurs.
2. Concentrate on decreasing that sense of urgency through a combination of rapid successive pelvic muscle contractions, distraction (maybe solve maths puzzles in your head!) and relaxation techniques (such as deep breathing).
3. After controlling the sense of urgency, walk slowly to the bathroom and let that pee out.
4. You have this under control? Awesome, now start to extend the time that you can delay your actual pee. Go for 30 or even 60 minutes if you can.
5. Continue this process until you only need to pee every three to four hours without incontinence.

Do pelvic floor exercises (with or without physiotherapy)

Strengthening the pelvic floor will help with stress incontinence. Here's how you do it:

1. The hardest part is working out which muscles are your pelvic floor muscles. You can't see them, so we go by feel. In your head, try to squeeze in a pee and stop yourself from peeing your pants. These are

the muscles you want to exercise; not so much your bottom, your thighs or your belly. If you're not sure, go to the toilet, start weeing and try to stop the flow. (I can't remember the last time I was able to actually do that!) There: those are the muscles to clench and tighten.

2. Start by clenching for two to three seconds, relaxing for five and doing this five times in a row. Three times a day. Then go for holding for longer: five and then maybe even 10 seconds, relaxing for 10 seconds, 10 times. You can do this twice a day. I'm not at 10 yet so I'll keep you posted!

3. Don't hold your breath. Keep breathing while you do your exercises.

4. Do this when you are doing something mundane and routine such as sitting in traffic.

It might take a while to tell they are working, but ideally you will notice four things:

- You have a longer time between bathroom visits.
- You have fewer 'accidents'.
- You can hold the contractions longer, or do more repetitions.
- You have fewer wet, smelly underpants.

Dr Dean Conrad, a Sydney-based gynaecologist with a special interest in urogynaecology and menopause, told me that he sees gym junkies whose every muscle is toned as a steel rod . . . except their pelvic floor. It turns out that doing pelvic floor exercises is hard and even exercise gurus struggle. So he always recommends at least a couple trips to a pelvic floor specialist physiotherapist to make sure your technique is good. 'With targeted physiotherapy alone, 50 per cent of stress incontinence can be cured or made significantly better,' he says.

Try vaginal oestrogen
Given this is the same oestrogen you'd be prescribed for sexual problems and vaginal dryness, you might be on this anyway. But studies do show less incontinence for women prescribed this therapy.

Weirdly, there is some evidence from trials that taking HRT by patches or orally actually makes urine incontinence worse! Nobody I've spoken to can explain it. Plus none of my patients has ever reported this to me; quite the opposite, actually. But, given the studies are there, I think the bottom line is: don't take HRT for the sake of your bladder!

Medication

A whole range of medications is available for urge incontinence. These include Solifenacin, Mirabegron, Trospium, Oxybutynin (tablets or patches) and Tolterodine. These are antispasmodics that decrease bladder activity by inhibiting contraction of the smooth muscle wall surrounding the bladder. They tend to have some side effects such as dry mouth and constipation. We have great short- and long-term data about the efficacy of these, especially Solifenacin, from numerous high-reliability clinical trials. Solifenacin has a pretty reasonable side effect profile, too. But it's an expensive option.

Botox for the bladder

Yes, for the bladder! Botox (Botulinum toxin), once known only as a life-threatening toxin from a nasty bacterium, has gone through a transformation, emerging as a powerful drug that temporarily paralyses muscles around the area it is injected. Botox is known for its popular use to paralyse the facial muscles, getting rid of frown lines. But it can do wonders for the bladder, too. It can be injected into the muscles at the base of the bladder, either in the specialist's rooms after some local anaesthetic, or under general anaesthetic. It starts to work in a few days, with full effect seven to 10 days later, and it needs to be done every six to 12 months.

The results are pretty impressive: in the biggest analysis of studies to date, between 42 and 87 per cent of patients returned to complete continence after treatment. Plus there was a 40–60 per cent decrease in complaints about frequently needing to pee and a 35–65 per cent increase in quality of life. And don't forget these studies were done in women who had tried everything short of surgery and failed. What we now know, having used it for a while, is that permanent changes in the bladder muscles can happen after repetitive treatment.

Sadly, a small percentage of patients who have lots of treatments with botulinum toxin will eventually become resistant to Botox.

Surgery

When you've tried all the options we've discussed above and urinary incontinence continues to disrupt your life, surgery might be an option. While there is no denying that surgery is more invasive and has a higher risk of complications than other therapies, it can also provide a long-term solution in severe cases when nothing else works. The type of surgery you would have would really depend on an accurate diagnosis, which is where urodynamic studies are essential. Surgery is better for stress than urge incontinence.

The most popular technique these days is the colposuspension technique. Most of my patients get a Burch colposuspension, which is just the specific technique used. Done by keyhole surgery, the urethra adjacent to the bladder is restored to its normal position and then stitched into place on either side. These stitches keep the bladder neck in place and help support the urethra.

In a sling procedure, strips of synthetic mesh (or sometimes a graft of your own tissue from the buttock or thigh) are used to make a kind of sling that supports the top of the bladder and the urethra. The sling helps keep the bladder neck closed when you jump, cough or sneeze, which hopefully prevents the leakage of urine. There is a lot of negative sentiment out there about synthetic mesh. Firstly, there is a small (less than 5 per cent) risk that the mesh will erode through the vaginal tissue — there are lots of lawsuits pending about this. Infection, bladder damage and chronic pain can also happen with the use of synthetic mesh.

No surgery is without risks, so chat to your doctor about what will work best for you.

Was that a wee, or are you just pleased to see me?

OK ladies, you're feeling in the mood, you have sex and, at the end, you're not sure what fluid is what and you think there might be some wee leakage involved. You felt as if you needed to wee during sex, or you just cannot be sure. Let me decode this for you. Weeing during an orgasm is a classic symptom of urge incontinence that we don't talk about. Yes it does happen. It's unlikely to be a full urination (around 100ml), but just leakage. It's still embarrassing and awkward, especially if it means you can only have sex in the shower or need to have sex on a towel. You will rarely have this happen in isolation and you will hopefully be getting some help for this problem anyway.

The other type of incontinence is the urge to wee or actually weeing *during* sex, pretty much as soon as the erect penis enters the vagina. This is a symptom of bladder prolapse. It often comes with a bit of stress incontinence as a symptom. It happens because the erect penis basically straightens out the vagina — that changes the pressure on your bladder and allows the urethra to open and let urine escape. If it doesn't worry you, great; but if that is beyond horrific and interfering with your love life, get a referral to a urogynaecologist for options.

How do you prevent UTIs after menopause?

I do need to mention that UTIs after menopause are *not* the way you remember from your twenties — the burning, stinging urine and the frequent trips to the loo only to pass a tiny dribble. In women approaching and after menopause, urine infections are often more subtle. You can have almost no symptoms other than feeling vaguely unwell. Or having smelly urine. Or your incontinence getting worse. Or all of those. Hence they can be missed and untreated, occasionally ending as a kidney infection that can land you in hospital. As a doctor, I was never told this. I learned the old-fashioned textbook version of bladder infections. It was only as my patients presented with vague, non-specific symptoms (for example, tired and nauseous) and mentioned an offensive-smelling either 'vaginal discharge' or urine (they often couldn't tell which) and I started checking, that the penny dropped. The way urine infections work in older women is *different*. On the plus side, keeping it in mind and testing for it gives rapid relief through antibiotics.

Here is my advice:

- Just keep urine infections in the back of your mind. If you get vague symptoms and an increase in incontinence or change in the smell of your urine, check in with your doctor sooner rather than later.

- Keep on drinking fluids. Lots of my patients, when faced with incontinence plus work or a party, just cut out the fluids. Being well hydrated helps prevent worsening UTIs.

- Travel (from a weekender to overseas) with antibiotics on you. Just in case.

This might shock you but if you get any more than *two* bladder infections in a six-month period, or three in 12 months, you have 'recurrent urinary tract infections'. Are you horrified? I'm guessing there are a lot of you who had no idea that is not normal and needs to be addressed. And, given that being a women over 55 years with a single UTI, you have a 53 per cent chance of getting a second infection within a year, even getting one is not a good thing.

Recent transition to menopause, having urinary incontinence, and a history of UTIs before menopause are all risks for recurrent UTI. I'm totally screwed. I don't want to gross you out too much but it is faecal bugs such as *E. coli* that are the primary villains involved in causing UTIs. They spread from the rectum to vagina (which is a pretty short hop) and from there travel up the urinary tract. A vagina that is unhealthy is a welcome landing spot for *E. coli*. Ideally the vagina should be acidic (with a *low* pH) and full of protective lactobacilli. A vagina that is too alkaline is not well equipped to repel the invading bacteria. The changing chemistry of the menopausal vagina is a special interest of mine.

Recurrent UTI affects one in five of us after menopause. To beat it you need a multi-pronged attack:

- Stay well hydrated. That's 2 litres of fluid a day for women. More if you're sweating because it's hot, you're flushing or you're exercising.

- Stay in a healthy weight range (I know: easier said than done). Being overweight or obese ups your risk of recurrent UTI.

- Always do a wee after sex. It mattered before menopause and it still matters now.

- Always take care to wipe front to back. (You don't need to give the *E. coli* from your rectum a free ride to the vagina!)

- Manage your constipation. Large amounts of poo in your large bowel can stop the bladder emptying well, which makes you more prone to UTIs.

- Manage your diabetes, if you have it. Poorly controlled diabetes can have the double-barrelled disadvantage of supplying a steady stream of sugar to hungry bacteria as well as a lowered immune system function. Poorly controlled diabetes also makes you more likely to get a complication such as a kidney infection.

Low-dose antibiotics

Because the cause of UTIs is bacteria, doctors often start treatment with antibiotics. Low-dose antibiotics acting as prophylaxis (prevention) are very effective; in fact, studies show they reduce the number of infections by a whopping 85 per cent. We use a low nightly dose that hits the sweet spot between enough antibiotics in the urine to kill the UTI-causing-bacteria, without the risk of resistance in the bowel flora — critical because the source of the offending bugs is the bowel. The big issue we are cautious about is breeding resistance to antibiotics — not only in you but in the wider community. So, many of us (me included) are keen to look at alternatives to antibiotics.

If you're sexually active, and you only get a UTI after sexual intercourse, your doctor can prescribe an antibiotic to take immediately after sex (that's just a one-off pill, not a course). A very small, prospective, placebo-controlled trial of healthy premenopausal women with a history of recurrent UTI received either a single dose of trimethoprim-sulfamethoxazole antibiotic after each occasion they had sex, or placebo used the same way. Nine out of the 11 women who took the placebo got a UTI, compared with two out of the 16 patients who took the antibiotic. It didn't matter how often or rarely the women actually had sex. Another study found this regimen is as effective as taking an antibiotic *every day*. I'd like a similar study on post- or perimenopausal women but these are the ones we have.

Vaginal oestrogen cream

Studies have found that vaginal oestrogen cream lowered vaginal pH from 5.5±0.7 to 3.6±1 (so from water to orange juice!), restored lactobacilli and helped prevent UTIs. Another prospective study showed that vaginal oestrogen reduced the incidence of UTIs in postmenopausal women to an average of half a UTI a year, compared to 5.9 episodes per year in women who took a placebo! Plus, after just one month of treatment, protective lactobacillus bacteria reappeared in 60 per cent of the women using vaginal oestrogen but in none of the placebo group. And the vaginal pH decreased from an average of 5.5 before treatment to an average of 3.6 after treatment. That is a seriously impressive treatment!

Sadly the same can't be said for standard HRT. Studies haven't found the same powerful benefits (of oestrogen directly into the vagina) from using transdermal or HRT pills when it comes to preventing UTIs. This seems kind of counterintuitive to me, but the studies are pretty conclusive. Where that leaves us is that you wouldn't go on HRT only to prevent recurrent UTI, but you *would* use vaginal oestrogen.

Methenamine hippurate

This over-the-counter tablet, made of a type of salt, acts as a kind of low-dose non-antibiotic antiseptic, specifically in the bladder. When it comes into contact with urine, it converts to formaldehyde, which helps kill bacteria. Taken twice a day, it seems to kill about 76 per cent of bacteria. I love this preparation because, in my experience as a doctor, it is really effective. But, because it is less widely studied, many doctors just bypass it. It has very few side effects other than being a pretty big pill that you need to take twice a day.

What about complementary and home remedies?

Cranberry

Wow! This has produced a mixed bag of studies. Some great results, some negative, and pretty much all *small* studies, which makes them less powerful. They range from drinking 50 to 250ml of pure juice a day, to powder, or tablets as well. There isn't a settled 'dose' for cranberry. The best I can say is that the jury is out on whether cranberry prevents UTIs. Drinking stacks of any fruit juice is a massive kilojoule load and, given the number of menopausal women battling bulges and expensive tooth issues, I'd go with cranberry supplements such as powder or tablets. Evidence is still lacking but enough small studies make them worth a shot. Zero Gwyneths.

Probiotics

The idea behind using probiotics in oral form is to rebalance the bacteria in the gut that seed the vagina. Again, the data is just *so* mixed! Studies for and against are confounded by the fact that the term 'probiotics' can mean varying numbers and concentrations of different probiotic bacteria. At this stage what we can say is that oral probiotics don't have any real evidence to support them. But if you swear by them, that's no drama. Zero Gwyneths.

There has been one fascinating study of weekly vaginal pessaries of *Lactobacillus crispatus*. This was used in a randomised controlled trial and it *halved* the number of UTIs in young women. It's pretty hard to find lactobacillus pessaries at a pharmacy or even online, but watch this space — they're coming!

Vitamin C

It's really popular, but the evidence to support this is a bit thin. Ascorbic acid (vitamin C) works to prevent urine infections by acidification of the urine. There was one study, done in young women, that found a weak link between vitamin C in the diet (not supplements) and a lower number of UTIs. In another study, 110 pregnant women were randomised to take either a supplement of iron and folic acid plus vitamin C daily or iron plus folic acid only. After three months the group with vitamin C in their supplement had far fewer UTIs. I am hoping for another, bigger study in postmenopausal women to get better data. I'm not aware of any of my patients using vitamin C as the only thing for prevention of recurrent UTI, so I just have no opinion. In a Petri dish, vitamin C limits the growth of bacteria in urine. And if you are using it and you think it's working, I have no problem with that. Zero Gwyneths.

D-mannose

D-mannose is a simple sugar found naturally in fruits and vegetables such as apples, broccoli, cranberries, oranges and peaches, among others. It actually can't be stored in the body and you wee it out pretty quickly.

D-mannose seems to bind to proteins on the *E. coli* bacterial walls, which prevents the bacteria from binding to the cells of the urinary tract. That sees the *E. coli* getting peed out instead of wreaking havoc in the bladder. In animals, D-mannose reduced bacterial 'colony-forming units' in the bladder fourfold.

Lots of trials have been done and, while the studies are small, the evidence for D-mannose is consistently pretty positive for preventing recurrent UTI. In fact, in the largest study to date, D-mannose was as good as antibiotics in that regard. There are two issues. The first is that this is a sugar and we see the same issues we warned about with cranberry. The second issue is that it might not be as good for non *E. coli* bacteria. While we definitely need more studies, at this stage I'd say D-mannose is safe, well tolerated and relatively inexpensive. Zero Gwyneths.

What is prolapse?

One of the most uncomfortable and awkward conditions to afflict many women after menopause is pelvic organ prolapse. If you've never heard about prolapse before, this could be pretty shocking. So, breathe . . . You have a few pelvic organs — such as the bladder, uterus, vagina and rectum — that sit on a sling of muscles stretching from the pubic bone to the coccyx. This is called the pelvic floor. Its role is to support the pelvic organs (it is woven around the vagina, urethra and rectum) and help you control your bladder and bowels. When the pelvic floor muscles relax, they allow urine to leave the bladder via the urethra and the pee comes out. When they contract, they close off the lower urethra, squeezing any remaining urine back up into the bladder.

Like any muscles, those of the pelvic floor weaken over time. Menopause definitely accelerates the process, which is worsened by vaginal delivery during childbirth and being overweight, as well as coughing fits.

A family history of prolapse also ups your risk, and chronic constipation that makes you frequently strain to poo is also a big contributor.

In prolapse, the pelvic organs *can* hang down into, and even bulge out of, the vagina. (My nana told me that her mother's uterus 'fell out' after delivering her fourteenth child.) Prolapse is super common. In fact, while it is only reported in 5 per cent of 60- to 69-year-old women, if a doctor examines you, some degree of prolapse is present in 41–50 per cent of women. Only 10 per cent or less of older women report any symptoms. So, what are those symptoms? You might feel a lump in the vagina, especially if you've been walking around for ages or exercising. Or you could just have a feeling of pressure in the pelvis, constipation, problems with weeing (getting a decent flow going), painful sex or even just a slow leak of urine.

Prolapse comes in four flavours: a cystocoele (when the bladder prolapses), uterine prolapse, vaginal prolapse (when the walls of the vagina sort of collapse inwards) and rectal prolapse (or rectocoele).

How do I get rid of it?

You don't necessarily need to. Gynaecologist Dr Dean Conrad says: 'If you don't have symptoms, in my book you don't have prolapse and you don't need treatment.' But, if you *do* have symptoms, we'd start with the easy stuff. Given that coughing, constipation and excess weight all put pressure on your pelvic floor, it's a good idea to address all of those in the same way as we advised for incontinence.

In the early stages, simply strengthening your pelvic floor (see pages 101–2) can help for mild to moderate prolapse of any kind, and can work pretty well in just three weeks. The exercises are better for 'front' prolapses (think bladder not rectal) and only work if you haven't had previous pelvic floor surgery.

If that doesn't work completely, pessaries would be our next step. Pessaries in this context are little cubes, rings or saucer-shaped plugs made of rubber or silicone. They are inserted into the vagina and literally add another level of support. These are still used in urogynaecology clinics all over the world. You can get DIY ones that you remove, clean and reinsert yourself, or you can have them put in by your doctor, and changed by your doctor every six weeks. We tend to keep those for much more elderly ladies who'd struggle with the whole DIY thing. While, for many women, these are preferable to surgery, they're not without issues. Not only can they irritate the vagina, but they can also cause pain, bleeding and even pressure sores. Pessaries can also lead to problems with bowel movements. Plus, you often can't have sex with them inside.

Surgery

Surgery is the remedy of last resort, if all else fails. Assuming your prolapse is making you pretty miserable, you would chat to a gynaecologist or urogynaecologist. You shouldn't make the surgical choice easily; for a start, there is absolutely no guarantee that this surgery will relieve all of your symptoms. Plus, there's always some risk of side effects such as vagina pain during intercourse, pelvic pain or worsening urinary incontinence.

You can opt for reconstructive surgery, which basically aims to restore the pelvic organs to their original position. These days, that is mostly done laparoscopically (via keyhole surgery). I'm not going to go into the various surgical techniques — they would be something you'd discuss with your specialist. As a very last resort, there is surgery in which the vagina is basically closed up so that nothing falls out of it (permanently taking the vagina out of action sexually).

A word on 'mesh' . . . This has been a really controversial subject since its use, in some types of surgery, caused chronic pain — it basically came out of place and eroded the vaginal wall. It was banned by the Food and Drug Administration (FDA) in the US for use in vaginal prolapse in 2019. So what is it, and what do you need to know about it?

Mesh is flexible, much like cloth, about 5mm thick and can be cut and tailored to fit your own pelvis. When used for bladder prolapse, it is placed about halfway along the 3cm urethra that takes urine from the bladder to the vulva. It's been used for 20 years for this purpose, with great data to support its efficacy and safety. It has an 'erosion rate' (when the mesh pops through the tissue) of 1 per cent. That's admittedly a very small risk. However, when used for vaginal prolapse, we saw erosion rates much higher — up to 20 per cent — which are unacceptable.

You will see Facebook pages dedicated to lawsuits against mesh, as well as calls for it to be banned in other jurisdictions. There are other surgeries for prolapse but their data is less established because they're newer. If you have a prolapse that has symptoms, get a referral to a specialist urogynaecologist and at least consider your options.

YOUR VAGINA AND BLADDER
THE BOTTOM LINE

Sisters, if some of us are talking about hot flushes, next to none of us are talking about the impact of menopause on our genitals, our bladders and our pelvic floors. We know the impact is huge. We also know that time is often a healer of hot flushes, but that's not the case with Genitourinary Syndrome of Menopause. It persists. And gets worse.

And the longer you delay getting treatment, the less likely it is to get fixed. We have options — really good options — for treating it.

Please find a doctor who will listen to you and discuss your options, so you can make the right decisions for your body.

CHAPTER 5

SOMEBODY BURNT DOWN MY HAPPY PLACE

A book about a positive menopause journey wouldn't be complete without looking at your emotional and spiritual wellbeing at this time. I am a fierce advocate for mental health: for my patients, friends and family, and for myself. I listen to endless podcasts on happiness and spirituality; I watch TED Talks and read (and now listen) to all of the top-selling books by gurus such as Gretchen Rubin, Eckhart Tolle and Spencer Johnson. I am fiercely protective of my medical students' spiritual and mental health, and let them know that my priority for our term is their emotional wellbeing. I protect my own, too; often gently but firmly pushing back against the demands of others that would cannibalise my time and happiness. So here, I want to dive into the subject of mental health, both for those with a diagnosable mental health issue (where the research is deeper) and those who just want to have a happier menopause journey.

Why do I feel like my hormones rule my brain?

It's a thing. To start with, the 'fairer sex' is more prone to depression than our brutish brothers. Depression is almost twice as common in women as in men (21 versus 12.7 per cent). And depression tends to last longer, recur more often, and be more severe and disabling for women than for men. And, if you suspected it, you're right: it gets worse around menopause time.

Many women already know that there is a huge neurobiological link between our hormones and our mood and behaviour. Many have experienced the dreaded premenstrual syndrome (PMS) or had our periods get out of whack when we're under a lot of stress. For that we can blame the effect of our hormones on the temporal lobes on either side of our brains.

Specifically, it is in the inner or medial portions of the temporal lobe where our emotions and our hormones come together and wreak havoc; it is where the temporal lobe houses the hippocampus and the amygdala. These are two important parts of the limbic system, a group of interconnected parts of the brain that sort through our emotions and allocate the right emotion to certain problems or situations. Your hippocampus sorts out your short-term memory, while the amygdala is where emotional relevance is mapped onto our memories. For example, if you are bitten by a dog, you might experience fear next time you see a dog. That is because your amygdala and hippocampus have colluded, with memory and emotion, to keep you safe and protect you from getting too close to dangerous dogs.

And the limbic system is the part of the brain that contains *most* of its oestrogen and progesterone receptors, making it most sensitive to hormonal swings.

The limbic system is also connected to two other vital parts of the brain (see Chapter 2, Meet your hormones), the hypothalamus and pituitary gland, which produce some of our female hormones. At times of stress, the amygdala and hippocampus can work together to shut down the sex hormones produced by the pituitary and hypothalamus, making your periods go haywire and stopping ovulation, or at least making it sporadic. This is obviously your body's way of stopping you getting pregnant at a tumultuous time — when the stress settles down and the hippocampus and amygdala work out that things are normal again, your hormones should right themselves.

Let's look at the specific actions of oestrogen and progesterone on your brain and go into some more detail about how your female hormones affect your brain and mood.

Oestrogen — the feel-good hormone

Oestrogen activates the oestrogen receptors that are on every cell in the brain to a greater or lesser degree. It increases the levels of the feel-good brain chemical, serotonin, and at the same time increases the number of serotonin receptors in the brain, meaning not only will you have more feel-good chemicals, but they will work more effectively as well. In addition, the enzyme tryptophan hydroxylase-2 (TpH2) converts the amino acid tryptophan into serotonin. Oestrogen increases the amount of serotonin in the brain. After menopause, the blood levels of serotonin decrease by about 50 per cent.

Oestrogen also affects the way another couple of feel-good neurotransmitters work in the brain. It increases amounts of noradrenaline (the target of many antidepressants) and decreases the brain activity of monoamine oxidase (MAO). MAO is a real downer in your brain; it breaks down your brain's feel-good serotonin and noradrenaline. More MAO = misery. MAO-inhibitors are also used as antidepressants.

So it should be no surprise that oestrogen, which is known to be an antidepressant in the lab situation, was once used as an antidepressant treatment. Think about postnatal depression, when there is a sudden fall off in oestrogen after the high levels of pregnancy. Professor John Eden, Head of the Sydney Menopause Centre at Royal Hospital for Women, told me that oestrogen used to be a treatment for bipolar disorder, major depression and schizophrenia. 'It worked,' he told me, but the side effects (especially in men) made it an unacceptable therapy; as specific antidepressants became available on the market, it was dropped altogether.

But don't be tempted to overdose on it. Too much oestrogen can be too much of a good thing; too much oestrogen not counterbalanced by progesterone can make you feel very anxious. In extreme situations, it can even induce seizures.

Progesterone — the chill-out hormone

Calming the situation is oestrogen's natural partner, progesterone. Studies have shown progesterone is a natural anti-anxiety chemical, not directly but because of its breakdown product, allopregnanolone. Allopregnanolone works via the neurotransmitter GABA, which is effectively an inbuilt tranquilliser.

Progesterone also seems to have a role as the maintenance guy in your brain. For example, after brain injury, progesterone appears to protect or rebuild the blood–brain barrier and reduce inflammation in the brain.

I haven't even reached menopause yet — so why do I feel depressed?

After perimenopause, once you do reach the other side of the rainbow (menopause proper), there might not be a pot of gold, but it could feel like it because the rate of depression actually decreases. The enormous Penn Ovarian Aging Study confirmed that it's the road *to* menopause that is linked to depression; life after established menopause is blessedly less prone to the Black Dog. And a large study published in the *British Medical Journal* found that one in three perimenopausal women had severe psychological symptoms, compared to one in four who had severe physical symptoms such as severe hot flushes.

Women with no history of anxiety are twice as likely to develop anxiety in perimenopause and very early menopause as at any other time in their life. And two to four times as likely to develop depression. That's going to see a whole heap of women suddenly saddled with a mental health diagnosis. I'm convinced that hormone changes play a massive role.

We think the problem in perimenopause is the wildly fluctuating hormone levels from day to day that trigger mood problems. In contrast, menopausal women have lower, but stable, oestrogen and progesterone levels.

Can we blame our hormones then?

Let's say that it's not *all* about hormone levels.

When scientists measure hormone levels in perimenopausal or postmenopausal women with depression, no abnormal levels are found compared to women at the same life stage who do not have a mental health problem.

Doctors have concluded that there is a group of women who are particularly sensitive to hormonal fluctuations. This group can be picked early; they tend to have either a history of mood disorders or PMS and/or post-partum anxiety or depression. So it is hormones plus maybe your genes combined that conspire to make menopause a moody time for some women. And, besides hormones and genes, there are some other culprits.

Hot flushes are bitches
Women with hot flushes are more likely to get mood problems than women without. It could be the lack of sleep. Could it also be that wild hormone swings cause both?

Alcohol
For some weird reason, research shows a spike in drinking and, to a lesser extent, smoking around menopause transition. Cause or effect? We still don't know.

Stress
Mood problems during perimenopause are more common in women with relatively low levels of education. Researchers have generally linked low levels of education with low socio-economic status and other stressors. Having no partner, or a partner you don't have a great relationship with, are also risk factors for mood problems at this time.

In studies, there are three major culprits for stress and menopausal depression: being sick (or having a family member or close friend who is sick); caring for aging parents; and changes in employment. Given how common these are as you start to get a bit older, no wonder it's such a common problem around menopause.

Then there are the psychological and social factors that happen around this time in your life:

- Change in the child-bearing role. A loss of fertility might be associated with the loss of an essential meaning of life, especially if you never had a child but wanted one.

- Empty-nest syndrome. I have to mention it as the research shows it's a factor, but I can't relate to this one myself. Surveys show that women whose children have moved out of home report more happiness and enjoyment in life than others. I miss my kids terribly, but life is certainly much easier now!

- Societal value of youth. In societies where age is valued, women tend to report fewer symptoms of menopause transition. I find that fascinating.

What happens after menopause?

When we observe women with depression during menopause transition, on the whole once they're on the other side of menopause, assuming no treatment, they can broadly fall into two groups. There are those who didn't have anxiety or depression before; their symptoms get better over time and generally by age 55 they're back to normal. (I'm not saying no depression or anxiety, but no spike in symptoms either — just an average risk.) Sadly, for the second group — women who have had anxiety or depression before but then spiral downwards in their mood during menopause transition — there is a worse prognosis and they are more likely to stay depressed for longer.

Therapies should always be tailored specifically to the woman by your health-care team, so I'm only going to go briefly through management options for anxiety and depression, specifically with a nod to menopause. There are entire books that deal with this. Let's just call it a helicopter view of your options so you can make an informed choice.

Can we treat depression with lifestyle changes?

For severe depression, overhauling your lifestyle is simply not the place to start. If you have such a severe mood disorder that you can't function at home or at work, you need urgent medical help. But if your depression and/or anxiety is mild to moderate, we will always try to manage your lifestyle first. Often making a few key changes is enough to turn the ship around.

These are my tips for handling stress and mild anxiety and depression. Some come from studies, most come from me!

Get some sleep

I have so many patients who come to see me in the middle of a crisis. They're almost ready to sign up for antidepressants — anything that will stop them feeling so bad. In 100 per cent of cases, assuming my patient is safe and neither suicidal nor homicidal, the first step is to get her sleep sorted. After all, Amnesty International has listed sleep deprivation as a form of torture and points out that it is illegal under the Universal Declaration of Human Rights. It always staggers me the number of people who put up with this sort of cruel, inhuman punishment, night in night out, without getting help. Step one of managing all mental health issues, from stress to depression and anxiety, is to sort out your sleep. Turn immediately to Chapter 6 for help with that.

Exercise

People who exercise have better mental health. For couch potatoes who suffer anxiety or depression, starting to exercise will improve your lot. We're still trying to get our heads around exactly why. We think that exercise positively affects your serotonin and GABA receptors. Exercise also helps the quality of your slow-wave sleep, improves your coping ability (or at least your perception of your ability to cope with stresses) and changes how much you focus on and obsess about things that worry you. How much exercise? Do what you can. There's no consensus yet, but 30 minutes a day seems reasonable. Most people can fit that into their lives.

Fix your food, fix your mood

Feeling down in the dumps makes you crave comfort foods. Feel too exhausted to stand and chop fresh veggies for dinner? And there is the ultimate Catch 22 . . . because eating crap foods not only makes you feel stuffed and sluggish in the bowels, but it also makes you tired and even more anxious and depressed. We now have multiple studies that show a diet with lots of junk food, soft drinks and added sugars can cause depressive symptoms.

The more research is done about the connection between your food and your mood, the more convinced we are of the link. We now know for example that roughly 95 per cent of your serotonin is produced by nerve cells that line your gastrointestinal tract. So the inner workings of your digestive system don't just help you digest food, but also impact on your emotions. Driving much of the function of the nerve cells that line your gut are the trillions of 'good' bacteria that make up your intestinal microbiome. We are only just starting to understand how important these microorganisms actually are. They not only protect the lining of your intestines by creating a barrier against toxins and 'bad' bacteria, they are also anti-inflammatory. They also influence the absorption of various nutrients from your food and activate neural pathways that travel directly between the gut and the brain. But change your diet and you will change the bacteria in your microbiome.

So which diet is best? Evidence is mounting. Studies have compared 'traditional' diets, such as the Mediterranean diet and the Japanese diet, to a typical 'Western' diet. They show that, quite apart from the substantial health benefits, the risk of depression is 25–35 per cent lower in those who eat one of these traditional diets. Not too much of a surprise really. For a start, traditional diets tend to be high in vegetables, fruits, unprocessed grains and fish and seafood. And they contain only modest amounts of lean meats and dairy. They also tend to have no processed snacks or added sugars, which are a big feature of any modern Western diet.

There is one fad food group that has been proposed to reduced anxiety and depression. I'm talking about fermented foods. Fermented foods have been exposed to apparently beneficial bacteria called lactobacilli. The bacteria feed on the natural sugars in the food, converting them to acid. Think foods such as kimchi, sauerkraut, kefir and yoghurt — but also the uber-cool kombucha and cafe-friendly sourdough bread. While some 'traditional diets' are high in fermented foods, there's no hard evidence they improve mental health on their own. So I would say if you like them, go for it. But if you don't, don't force them on yourself.

Probiotics

Given the influence we know the gut microbiome has on your risk of anxiety and depression, no wonder there is so much interest in the potential role for probiotics to boost mental health. So researchers in the US conducted a review of all the medical studies on probiotic use to treat anxiety and depression. They published it in the *Annals of General Psychiatry*. (None of the studies were much chop, mind you, having fairly small numbers of patients, and not including much follow-up over time.) The results of these studies were mixed. Some reported mild benefits in taking probiotics for anxiety or depression, while other studies showed they didn't help. The authors concluded that there simply isn't enough evidence to advocate the use of probiotics for these mental health conditions. Oh well, keep the studies coming!

Chewing gum

That sounds nutty, right? But studies have shown that chewing gum not only enhances your concentration, but makes you feel happier, too. Chewing gum made these study subjects significantly more alert and they reported less stress while doing their tasks. Plus, they had lower levels of salivary cortisol. And apparently their tasks were performed better. I know what I will be doing the next time a complex patient comes in for a tricky diagnosis!

Stand up straight!

Depressed people often slouch, but is slouching the cause or the effect of depression? A few studies have sought to prove that standing up straight and fixing your posture can improve your mood. Using physiotherapists armed with physio tape to fix the posture of depressed slouchers, the researchers found that better posture improved mood, reduced tiredness and stopped people focusing on themselves. It's not the only study to find this link between better posture (sitting and standing) and better mood. So tuck in your tummy, throw your shoulders back and hold your head high. Or seek the help of a physiotherapist.

What are the psychological therapies?

If you have been diagnosed with depression or anxiety and someone writes you a prescription for medication without first trying to give your brain some psychological help to manage your symptoms, walk away now. Seeing a clinical psychologist or counsellor for strategies and tools to help manage your emotions is an essential part of getting well.

I have many patients who are very resistant to having therapy. 'I've tried it, it doesn't work.' My analogy is this: you cannot join the gym and then give up a week later because you aren't running a marathon yet. It takes time and practice. You also need to find the right person. I refer to a few psychologists and I always make sure I tailor the therapist to my patient's needs and desires on this journey.

For others, the issue is price. I cannot argue with this; it is quite an investment. But, in some ways, I think you can't afford *not* to do it. After all, what is life about? There are now free online therapy courses that are a great option for those who simply cannot afford face-to-face consultations. Here are some of the psychological therapies used by many doctors and psychologists.

Meditation

Meditation can be described as a variety of mind-regulation practices that focus on training your attention and awareness. Broadly speaking, there are two main types of meditation. The first is concentrative meditation, where you concentrate on something (such as a particular phrase). The second is mindfulness meditation, which involves a broader awareness and maintaining a moment-by-moment mindfulness of thoughts, feelings, bodily sensations and even your environment, through a gentle, non-judgemental lens.

So, lots of people hear the word meditation and think flowing robes, panpipes and incense, or people who are so chilled anyway that they practically meditate through life. I hear it all the time: 'I've tried meditating and I can't do it!' But meditation doesn't need to be oms and chakras and lotus positions. You can do a quick form of mindfulness meditation that really, really works. A 2014 study showed that mindfulness meditation led to some benefits and appeared to provide as much relief from some anxiety and depression symptoms as other studies have shown from antidepressants.

One of the problems in understanding the effectiveness of meditation is that there is no standard way to do it. The mindful meditation routine that works for me is:

1. Sit on a comfortable chair. Push your bottom right back in the chair. Make sure your feet are resting gently on the ground, equally weighted.
2. Gently close your eyes. Don't scrunch your eyelids up; just rest them very gently together.
3. Relax your feet, resting them gently on the floor.
4. Relax your thighs, letting them fall into the chair.
5. Let your tummy blob out, no holding it all in!
6. Let your shoulders drop. Let your hands rest comfortably in your lap.
7. Relax your brow. Unclench your jaw.
8. Take a long, slow breath in through your nose and out again, through your nose.
9. As you breathe, focus all your mind on the way the air feels cooler and sharper going in, and warmer and softer going out.
10. Just focus on the way the breath feels on the tip of your nose.
11. If your mind wanders, imagine yourself scooping your thoughts back and placing them gently on the tip of your nose.
12. Slowly focus on three distinct things you can hear. Just list them slowly in your head. It might be the traffic outside, the hum of a computer, a voice in the distance.
13. Keep breathing.
14. Slowly focus on three distinct things you can feel. Just list them slowly in your head. It might be the way your back feels against the chair, the way your left hand feels against your left thigh . . .

The secret is to practise. Start with 20 minutes a day — this number is highly unscientific. It's my number. If you can only manage five minutes, do that! Once you are good at it and can switch your mind off quickly, you can do it whenever you want and whenever you need it most. And you can add in a five-minute meditation when you're feeling exhausted, if you can find a park bench or quiet spot to sit. If doing this alone seems just too much, try downloading a meditation app. While they don't have scientific rigour to prove they work, they're unlikely to lead you astray either.

Mindfulness

Mindfulness essentially gets you to be in the present and not worry obsessively about what was or might be (known as 'ruminating'). It is a way of thinking about the world around us that is broader than just meditation. As an example, look around the room and note down silently everything that is blue. Now close your eyes and recite them back to yourself. If I then asked you, without opening your eyes, to list the green things in the room, I think you'd struggle to name more than one or two. You were so intent on studying the blue objects that the green objects simply escaped your attention. The mind is like that — some of the loveliest, cutest, funniest, saddest and weirdest things can completely pass us by because we're focused on the tasks in front of us.

Mindfulness is one of the techniques used by psychologists to deal with people who are stressed, anxious or depressed. When you can't see the big picture of tranquillity and happiness, you might be able to put one together with tiny patches of happiness from your day. But you need to notice them and take them on board. The feeling of the sun on your face; the sound of children laughing; the smell of a fantastic coffee or cake shop; the look on your toddler's face when he stands on sand or laughs at Dora or Elmo. Those tiny moments can pass us by so quickly, barely penetrating the surface of our busy, crazy, stressed-out worlds. Don't let even one fly past without seizing it and making sure it sinks into your soul and adds a patch to your happiness quilt.

Unfortunately, bad feelings, thoughts and experiences tend to sink in and grip into our souls like fishing hooks. So, when a bad thought comes, allow it to emerge and then let it float away. Don't hold on to it: just imagine it, like a leaf floating down a river, passing through you instead of hooking into you. If you hold on to bad thoughts, they can damage you.

Are there herbal, or other, remedies that might help me?

The list of these is long, and I don't want to leave any out. So mosey your way through them all in case any are useful for you.

St John's wort

Also known as hypericum, this is a popular supplement for depression and anxiety. It has actually been trialled in menopause but for vague things such as 'symptoms of menopause', rather than depression and anxiety, and depression around menopause per se. The results have been reasonable. The standard dose is 300mg three times a day with meals. If you use it properly it's very safe with few nasty side effects (some minor tummy upsets and skin becoming more sensitive to sunlight so burning more easily). However, you should *never* take it without checking with your doctor first: it interacts with many medications, including the contraceptive pill, antidepressants and antihistamines. One Gwyneth.

Ginkgo biloba

When I was in China, this weird-looking herb (also known as maidenhair) was at the front of every pharmacy and traditional Chinese medicine shop. It is mostly used for dementia (see Chapter 8, The sharpest tool in the shed), but in one study of 107 patients specifically to look at anxiety, there were some pretty huge improvements from taking ginkgo, especially those on the higher dose (480mg). It's only one study, so not proof. Ginkgo is not cheap and it interacts with many medications and supplements, so tread carefully and run it by your GP or pharmacist first. One Gwyneth.

Magnesium supplements

Magnesium is a mineral found in foods such as dark green veggies, legumes, nuts and whole grains. Most healthy people have normal levels of magnesium, despite the fact that, at least in the US, studies consistently show that intake is inadequate. There are a couple of pretty poor-quality studies to link magnesium supplements with lower anxiety. If you're sleep deprived and are taking it to help you sleep, there might be some added benefit to your mood, too. Zero Gwyneths.

Passionflower

Some researchers believe that passionflower supplements may help treat anxiety and depression, as well as some types of pain, because they may increase levels of gamma-aminobutyric acid (GABA), a chemical the brain makes to help regulate mood.

There are a couple of (albeit tiny) randomised trials that compared passionflower with benzodiazepines for anxiety over a four-week period. In both studies, there were no significant differences between benzos and passionflower, and side effects were pretty similar. One small placebo-controlled trial of 182 people with anxiety disorder found passionflower thumped placebo on the Hamilton Anxiety Rating Scale (you guessed it: a measure of anxiety). These studies are too small to be 100 per cent sure, but there doesn't seem to be much downside. Zero Gwyneths.

Valerian root

Valerian is another herb that switches on the GABA receptors, which might be why it has been used as a treatment for insomnia and depression for a long time. Sadly, the results of the small number of trials done to assess it have been a bit of a bust. A Cochrane review of valerian for anxiety focused on a small four-week trial in 36 adults diagnosed with generalised anxiety disorder. These study subjects were randomised to take valerian, a benzo-diazepine or placebo. In the end, valerian and placebo yielded the same results. So, there's not enough evidence to get a thumbs up but it's well tolerated and there are no safety concerns. Zero Gwyneths.

5-hydroxy-tryptophan

This amino acid is the immediate precursor of serotonin and can be purchased as an over-the-counter dietary supplement in some countries. There are many poor-quality studies on the use of tryptophan and 5-hydroxy-tryptophan in depression. One study of 10 people found that tryptophan or 5-hydroxy-tryptophan *did* improve mood more than a placebo. Another trial of 24 sufferers of panic disorder found that 200mg of 5-hydroxy-tryptophan taken 90 minutes before a panic-inducing challenge significantly reduced anxiety compared to the placebo. But with such tiny studies, it's hard to know whether it's a winner or not. And it has not been tried in menopausal women specifically. In Australia and other countries, the sale of tryptophan is restricted. You can get low doses over the counter in pharmacies, but the higher doses are more difficult to obtain. I found lots of apparently high-dose products (500mg or even more) by searching through some online vitamin shops, but I couldn't see any oversight to make sure the quality of the product is decent. I think there are better supplements and treatments for you out there, so I wouldn't bother. Two Gwyneths.

Fish oil

Fish oil is a type of omega-3 fat, a polyunsaturated fatty acid. There are three different types of omega-3 fatty acids: alpha-linolenic acid (ALA); eicosapentaenoic acid (EPA); and docosahexaenoic acid (DHA). ALA is found mostly in walnuts, some seeds and some oils. EPA and DHA are found in oily fish, such as tuna and salmon, and eggs. ALA is converted into EPA and DHA by the body.

The rationale for its use in mental health disorders (not specifically menopause related) is threefold: research has shown that some people with depression have lower levels of omega-3 in their red blood cells. So it's possible that low omega-3 might contribute to depression. Secondly, countries with high fish consumption have lower rates of depression. And finally, there is emerging evidence that depression is caused by inflammation. And we think omega-3 may reduce inflammation.

So does it work? It sure looks that way! A meta-analysis of 11 trials found that omega-3 helped reduce depressive symptoms, especially in people who were taking antidepressant medications. It can interact with some medicines, so check in with your pharmacist or GP before starting, but given it is cheap and has relative few side effects, I think it's totally worth a shot. Zero Gwyneths.

Withania somnifera

This plant (also known as ashwagandha) has been touted in India as a treatment for everything from arthritis to attention deficit hyperactivity disorder, insomnia to tuberculosis, asthma to backache, Parkinson's disease to an underactive thyroid. Oh, and anxiety. If this were true, I could retire right now.

Am I going to have to eat my words? There is a double-blind, placebo-controlled study of ashwagandha happening as I write this in 39 patients with anxiety. It has stated that the people taking ashwagandha reported much less anxiety than those taking the placebo after six weeks. Plus, it caused no more adverse effects than the placebo. It does have quite a few interactions with medicines so check in with your GP or pharmacist before you start. I found ashwagandha online for a pretty cheap price, but can't verify that it contains what it says. But it might be worth a shot. One Gwyneth.

Lysine

This isn't a herb, but rather an amino acid, better known for fighting cold sores. Recent studies in animals have identified that lysine may influence neurotransmitters involved in stress and anxiety. In fact, lysine was shown in these studies to decrease the brain–gut response to stress as well as lowering blood-cortisol levels.

Researchers went to Syria (a place where stress and anxiety levels are undoubtedly through the roof). They added lysine supplements to wheat for three months and found that the amino acid reduced stress in women and anxiety in men. More research was done in Japan with people without a diagnosed anxiety disorder but who were experiencing some anxious symptoms. This randomised placebo-controlled trial confirmed that, in combination with another amino acid, arginine, there were lower feelings of anxiety together with lower salivary-cortisol levels.

So, there are not too many side effects or interactions, but enough evidence to give it a shot? Solid maybe. Zero Gwyneths.

Bach flower remedies

Bach flower remedies are a system of 38 flower extracts (including passionflower) developed by Dr Edward Bach in the 1930s. They are made by steeping fresh flowers in water in the sun for a few hours, then preserving the water with alcohol. I'm not sure how much flower is left in the 'remedy'. An example is Rescue Remedy, which is super popular and can be bought over the counter in pharmacies and health-food shops. How does it work? I'm straightening my face as I tell you that Bach flower remedies harness the plant's life-force energy, thus eliminating emotional imbalances. Really? Despite the highly suspect mechanism of action, a trial has actually been done! And it was a bomb. Ninety-eight people suffering with mental health conditions from anxiety disorders and depression to schizoaffective disorder were randomised to take either Rescue Remedy or a placebo for three days. There was no difference in anxiety symptoms between the two groups. Save your money. Two Gwyneths.

Homeopathy

I know it's popular, but seriously? This is what I'd term 'a crock'. Homeopathic remedies are made by diluting various substances with water and alcohol, and shaking them. This process is then repeated over and over until there is little or none of the original substance left. So . . . it's water and alcohol. The whole concept of homeopathy is based on the principle of 'like cures like'. The diluting and shaking is meant to simultaneously remove any harmful effects of the original substance, while the water retains the 'memory' of the substance. And that's not a joke.

And yet studies have been done. The only one specifically for anxiety was a trial of 44 adults with generalised anxiety disorder. It compared individually tailored homeopathic medicines with placebo for 10 weeks. I am happy to report that the people on homeopathy did not do worse than those on the placebo; in fact, the improvement from the placebo and the homeopathy were the same. Yet another reminder that the human mind is mysterious and that the placebo effect should not be discounted. One Gwyneth.

Negative ions into the air

This sounds like rubbish but seems to have some decent evidence. What we're talking about here are electrical devices called 'air ionisers' that produce negative air ions for your room. A negative air ion is an atom that has gained an electron and so has a negative charge. Meanwhile, a positive ion has lost an electron so has a positive charge. Both positive and negative ions are found naturally in the air; however, experts say, fresh air has more negative ions — they're produced by natural phenomena including lightning, ocean waves and waterfalls.

Treatment generally involves sitting in a room with the ioniser on for 30 minutes every morning for two to three weeks. This has the best evidence for depression that comes on in winter (seasonal affective disorder — SAD) when I guess we're naturally getting less fresh air. But studies on other forms of depression that run throughout the year look pretty positive, although it's early days. Regardless, using a high-density ioniser is more effective than using a low-density ioniser.

The machines do make ozone, so a 20–30 minute stint is plenty and make sure to air the room afterwards. Otherwise, the downside is just the cost. If you're going to invest in one, make sure to buy a high-density ioniser. It produces 2,700,000 ions per cubic centimetre, while a low-density one produces only 10,000 ions per cubic centimetre. One Gwyneth (weighing up the possible benefits against the expense and the ozone).

Kava

Go to the Pacific Islands and the kava drink (often part of a welcome ceremony) is everywhere. Made of a Pacific root vegetable soaked in water and kneaded, it was banned from import into Australia in 2007 because it is basically a sedative and has high abuse potential. In 2019 it was brought back — more for political than medical reasons. Regardless, let's check out its effects on anxiety. Exhibit A, have you ever been to Fiji? If so, have you ever met an indigenous Fijian with mental health issues? Me neither. I have been to a few kava ceremonies over the years and maybe it's because I'm a cheap drunk (or perhaps I'm representative of most people), but it pretty much knocked me out. After the most recent ceremony, in which the chief of a remote Fijian village personally made us kava, I had to co-run a medical clinic. That was tough!

There is science, too. A recent Cochrane review of placebo-controlled trials found 12 to review. The authors concluded that: 'Compared with placebo, kava extract is an effective symptomatic treatment for anxiety, although, at present, the size of the effect seems small.' What we don't know is how much to take and for how long.

Plus, kava has a few downsides. Herbal remedies that contain kava extract have been linked to irreversible liver damage. Long-term use has also been linked to everything from mood swings and apathy to shortness of breath. And it interacts with heaps of drugs. Bottom line, inconclusive . . . this one is not for the faint-hearted. Two Gwyneths.

Black cohosh

We already met this member of the buttercup family for hot flushes. If you remember, it contains a number of compounds that, in a Petri dish, mimic oestrogen. If you do a search of depression and anxiety in menopause, you'll get lots of results praising black cohosh as an effective remedy. The problem is, there are close to no studies that support this perspective.

There was one tiny prospective, placebo-controlled trial of 25 women, which didn't find black cohosh any better than the placebo. Another longer term and slightly larger study also failed to find a benefit. I just wouldn't bother. There are better things out there. Two Gwyneths.

What about antidepressant medication?

I have not put this first. I want to deal with this because, when nothing else works, your depression or anxiety is moderate to severe and symptoms are impacting on your quality of life, these medications can be lifesaving. But they're far from a panacea. They have significant side effects that you need to be aware of and they don't work for everyone. While, for many doctors, writing a prescription is the easiest thing to do, for me it is the final frontier and I don't prescribe them lightly.

The idea behind antidepressant medications is to increase the levels of feel-good neurotransmitters in the brain. Some target serotonin; others noradrenaline. Some newer ones even increase melatonin.

A 2018 meta-analysis looked at 522 trials of 21 antidepressants with over 100,000 people suffering moderate to severe depression. It found they were at least twice as effective as the placebo in every case. When they played effectiveness off against side-effect profile, they came up with their top five antidepressants: SSRIs Escitalopram, Paroxetine and Sertraline; and atypical antidepressants, Agomelatine and Mirtazapine. I will mention Venlafaxine here, because, while it didn't feature in this review, it is pretty effective for depression and also for managing hot flushes, so I use it in menopause sometimes to get a dual effect.

But you need to know a couple of things about antidepressants before you start. Low libido, weight gain, nausea, feeling tired and feeling like you're in an emotional straightjacket are all possible side effects. And there is a withdrawal syndrome. Stop them too quickly and you can get severe symptoms, from the famous 'brain zaps' to physical symptoms such as dizziness and flulike symptoms, insomnia, nausea and hot flushes. But worse, it can feel like the depression is coming back. To avoid this we stop them over about four weeks. Certain antidepressants are worse for this than others, so check in with your doctor. But, please, never just stop taking these drugs cold turkey.

And can HRT help depression?

The link between hot flushes and mood symptoms has been pretty well shown in many studies now. In fact, in one Aussie study of menopausal women, those with moderate to severe hot flushes were almost three times as likely to get moderate to severe depression as women with mild flushes. This was independent of job, weight, age, relationship and financial situation. Come on, surely this doesn't surprise you? The same severe hot flushes were linked to a higher likelihood of binge drinking and smoking, and ending up on some kind of mood medication. Fix the hot flushes; see Chapter 3, Baptism by fire.

Anecdotally, many women on HRT see a huge improvement in mood symptoms. Endocrinologists say the evidence for HRT is a tad sketchy but on balance it probably works.

The pill itself is also interesting here. In perimenopause, when mood problems are often at their worst, we often use the contraceptive pill instead of HRT because we're trying to regulate the cycle but HRT won't guarantee contraceptive effect. Dr Roisin Worsley of Jean Hailes for Women's Health in Melbourne did some fascinating work around different contraceptive pills and the rate of depression. Interestingly, even though Yaz — a low-dose pill containing the anti-androgen progestin drospirenone — is marketed specifically for PMS, women on drospirenone-containing pills had a higher risk of depression. In fact, Dr Worsley said she always avoids these pills in women with mood issues. She says she prefers contraceptive pills that contain oestradiol (instead of the more common ethinyl oestradiol). That's based on her clinical experience and not any studies: the studies simply haven't been done.

So where does that leave hormone therapies for depression during peri-menopause? The bottom line is that the pill is unlikely to work.

Kerry's story

Around six months ago I saw Kerry, a regular patient. Two years earlier, at age 48, she'd gone on a massive health kick. This was after being diagnosed with obesity, high blood pressure, a uterus full of polyps and fibroids that were giving her hell and resulted in a hysterectomy, plus a variety of other issues. She'd lost 40kg with a personal trainer and some major diet modifi-cations. She looked terrific, felt great and was sleeping well.

So when she came in, burst into tears and said, 'I just don't feel like me,' I was shocked. She told me that after running her first 11km community run a month earlier, she'd started getting anxiety attacks and palpitations. She was exhausted all the time, had aches and pains, and hadn't been to her trainer in a month — and she'd gained 8kg in a month! She was crying all the time and couldn't sleep. In all the years I had known her, Kerry had never had mood issues. She was always a pretty contented soul, even when her health had been in a bad place.

'Are you having hot flushes?' I asked her.

'Yes' she said. She'd put that all down to anxiety. I put it all down to menopause. With no uterus, and therefore no periods, she just hadn't been focusing on her hormone health.

I suggested a patch of oestradiol. Well, I didn't see her again until she came back the other day for a flu shot and another prescription for her patches. 'It took three days,' she told me. All her symptoms were gone. She's lost the 8kg she'd gained and a little more. She told me it was like that bad month is just a bad memory. I can't promise everyone will experience the dramatic benefits that Kerry did. But her story is not uncommon.

I'm not depressed; I'm just not that happy

You might not have depression per se, but just aspire to greater happiness overall. The field of 'positive psychology' has taken off over recent years with some amazing results. I certainly don't propose to be an expert in the field but I know that your level of happiness and satisfaction can now be measured. And that not being happy can affect your productivity at work, the quality of your relationships and your risk of a proper mental health disorder. I think you owe it to yourself to be the happiest possible version of you. I loved *The Happiness Project* by Gretchen Rubin; she takes the matter of her happiness pretty seriously. And I was able to benefit from much of her research and experimentation around improving her happiness.

I have collated a few ideas from gurus I interviewed for this book, from research into positive psychology, and my own personal favourites. These will hopefully help you combat stress, increase your happiness and transform your menopause journey.

Sue's story

One of my patients, Sue, was 48 and at peak perimenopause. She was a mess. Her job, the thing that had brought her pride, fulfilment and pleasure had overnight become a place of hurt, shame, fear and anxiety. She does amazing work caring for unfortunate people in our community. Many have complex mental health or drug and alcohol conditions. Her enormous heart had been poured into her clients and they loved her back. To her horror, she was called into a meeting and asked to sit on one side of a table facing her manager and two people from management she hardly knew. She discovered she was there to answer an allegation that she was overly familiar with her clients. To the point of being inappropriate. She was called on to explain her behaviour, and specific examples were provided. Sue was devastated. She burst into tears; she felt humiliated, defensive, embarrassed, hurt and ashamed. And within five minutes she felt angry.

Her critical colleague, the one who had submitted the complaint against her, was inexperienced, new and not great at her job, she told me. She was jealous, ineffectual and the clients didn't like her. She was trying to cause trouble for Sue in the one place that made her feel good about herself. As a single mum, Sue had struggled financially and without qualifications, it had taken a long time to find this role. One at which she felt she excelled. Now she was assailed by self-doubt. She couldn't sleep; she felt anxiety as she woke in the morning and got ready for work. She felt sick as she sat on the bus on the way to work. She became paranoid — who else was in on this ridiculous complaint? Her anger became focused on the colleague that she felt had wronged her. It took a while but she had to forgive her colleague.

Forgiveness is about *you* being able to let go of those destructive, negative, hurtful thoughts, not about condoning the behaviour of whoever has treated you badly. In many cases that person is getting on with their life and not giving you so much as a backwards glance. The only one suffering is you. Let that negative energy go and with it, regain your sense of self and become the more positive, optimistic person you deserve to be.

I always refer to that sort of hurt and negativity as the dog poo on your shoe. Stepping in it in the first place is a pain in the arse. But it's happened. Now it's up to you . . . You can either wipe it off your shoe or continue to tread it grudgingly through your house, getting it on your carpets. Do you want to carry that negativity you feel towards someone who has wronged you all the way through your life like that dog poo, ruining your meta-phorical carpets? Forgive them, and get it off your shoe.

You don't have to be naive. You don't have to resume a friendship with someone who doesn't deserve it, but you can be free from bitterness and negativity.

Ellen's story

Ellen came to see me about four months ago. At 50 and still having regular periods, she had started to develop some significant mental health symptoms she hadn't seen since the birth of her last child 16 years previously, when she suffered postnatal depression. She wasn't sleeping, and she was spending time in the bathroom at work in tears pretty much every day. Her boss seemed to have it in for her, she told me. She couldn't do anything right. She was missing deadlines and making mistakes. She'd had a formal 'warning' and was worried about losing her job. She would get a headache on the bus in to work and a feeling of dread in the pit of her stomach. It wasn't just at work — she was withdrawn at home and had stopped making arrangements with her husband or friends to go out. She'd not gone to the gym for over six months now. Worst of all, she'd started having fleeting thoughts of suicide. 'I'd never do it,' she told me. But I wasn't surprised that when we did a formal test called the DASS 21, her depression score was severe.

I did notice she'd put on weight, but was alarmed when we got her on the scales. It was a 16kg weight gain since I'd last weighed her a few years ago! She admitted her diet was bad. She'd leave home without breakfast, feeling too nauseous to eat; she'd have Coke, chips and chocolate during the day and couldn't be bothered cooking at night so the whole family had taken to getting home-delivery Thai or pizza unless her mum had dropped in a meal.

Her blood pressure was high and it turned out her blood-test results were horrible.

Here's what she didn't have: hot flushes, night sweats, heavy periods or aches and pains. But she's 50. So I'd bet my bottom dollar she's in perimenopause.

In Ellen's case, we didn't talk about hormone treatments. Even though she is clearly in a perimenopausal age group, the impetus to treat her severe depression trumped everything else.

There are many priorities for someone like Ellen: attending to her physical health, including her diet and lack of exercise, lowering her blood pressure, fixing her lack of sleep and managing her stress at work were top priorities (with the help of a counsellor). As was managing her depression. In her case, the first antidepressant medication we tried, which targeted her brain's serotonin levels, worked a treat.

Now we're doing the major task of overhauling her diet, really nailing her sleep and getting her to build exercise into her day. It's a bit 'two-steps-forward-one-step-back'. Anyone who tells you that it's easy is having you on. But Ellen is coping at work, hasn't cried in the bathroom for months now, is coping better with household tasks and last week she went out for a girls' night! She's slowly turning the ship around.

Switch loss to freedom

Highly respected clinical psychologist Jo Lamble has written a mountain of books on anxiety, depression, relationships and more. She's also my colleague and dear friend. So, of course, I chatted to her about stress, anxiety, depression-boosting and happiness during menopause. 'There's a group of women who have added stress because they're in that sandwich generation,' she said. 'But overwhelmingly it's about loss. Loss of fertility, loss of youth, loss of attractiveness, loss of femininity.' She says this can come packaged with fear about relationships. Women worry that their newly old and unattractive bodies will see their partners lose interest and wander elsewhere.

She focuses instead on turning that loss and fear into freedom. Liberated of the need to focus on our looks, women around menopause can focus instead on what is real: the people we are, the relationships we have, and a new sense of purpose. I recently spoke to a group of women aged around 50 and they were pumped about not caring about what anyone else thinks of them anymore. They were doing what was right for them and the people who meant most to them. Many, freed of having to be home to cook for kids and take them to various after-school activities, were now able to join a choir or book club, take up golf or learn a language. As Jo says, that's real freedom.

Feel gratitude

It is easy to spend masses of energy thinking about the things that are suboptimal in your life: great holidays that your friend has, but you can't afford; a colleague's job success that has evaded you. But those feelings wreak havoc on your mind and body. Gratitude is worth aiming for. Research shows that grateful people sleep better, are less depressed, feel more energetic, have more self-confidence and have less inflammation in their bodies. Researchers at the University of California, Berkeley also discovered that simple gratitude journalling, in addition to getting medical help, gave patients lower levels of inflammatory markers and increased heart-rate variability (HRV), a key indicator of heart health, than patients who received medical care alone.

It's time to focus on the good things that you have and reasons you are fortunate. If you are feeling stressed or a little down, I want you to grab a pen and paper right now and write down 10 things for which you are grateful. If your mind is in a bad space, that can be difficult. They can be as general as living in a free country, having an able body (if you do) or being able to afford food and clothing. Studies have found that being grateful is one of the most successful strategies to achieve real contentment and happiness, as well as better physical health.

If you've never been especially grateful, you can try a few things to get it going. Write a letter to someone to whom you are grateful. You don't have to send it — just writing the letter seems to help. Or try gratitude journalling. Studies have found that just writing down things for which you are grateful in your own scrapbook can give you better sleep, fewer symptoms of illness and more happiness. Finally, you can pray. I'm not especially religious, but prayer in its purest form is more about giving thanks than asking for things.

So, a couple of caveats about gratitude . . . There's no real evidence that these simple steps will give you any significant and permanent benefits. Gratitude doesn't instantly transform your mental health, but the Berkeley studies show that gratitude improves your mental health cumulatively over time.

Fake it till you make it

A month ago I saw Sarah. 'I need help,' she said. She'd been really stressed at work. Her responsibilities were piling up and yet her salary wasn't. In fact, there were so many retrenchments in her company each month that she was worried about losing her job if she pushed back against her escalating workload. And her new boss was horrible. He had gained a promotion she thought he wasn't equipped for and he managed his team by insulting everyone and generally being a dickhead. Sarah was a coiled-up spring of fear, stress and anxiety. And her family was copping it. She'd taken to 'letting it all out' when she got home. The week before this had culminated in her physically punching her partner during an argument, and her 17-year-old son announcing he was moving to his dad's and that he didn't want to hear from her for a bit. 'I can't do this,' she sobbed.

'Did hitting your partner help? Did you feel a bit better afterwards when you let it all out?' I asked.

'No,' she confessed. 'I think it made it worse.' Bingo. Many people assume that behaviour follows mood. I'm happy, therefore I sing to myself and smile. I'm angry, therefore I throw my phone against the wall. In fact, research tells us the opposite is true.

The way you behave actually shapes emotion. I know that sounds crazy but it's true. You feel sad *because* you cry, you feel angry *because* you lashed out. Research has shown that the fastest way to change the way you feel is to *change your behaviour*. If you want to feel happy, act like a happy person. And *most importantly*, if you don't want to be angry, don't act like an angry person. If you don't want to be afraid, don't act scared. You don't get to yell at anyone in your family. You don't get to 'let it all out', because there are no winners from that strategy.

Sarah and I negotiated a plan. Go in to work smiling, relax your shoulders, ditch the resting bitch face and say hello to everyone with a big, generous smile. Go home and get into comfy clothes, pop on some happy music and dance around the kitchen. Withdraw any permission you thought you had to 'let out' your negative emotions to your loved ones. That was seriously all it took for Sarah to feel better in two weeks. True story.

Smile

Put good energy out into the world. When I first met Daniel, my husband, I was a runner. A really bad runner, mind you. But I ran a lot. And I ended up with muscles so tight I felt like a lump of tightly constructed concrete. Weirdly enough, it was in my neck and shoulders that the muscle tightness was worst. Daniel, who is a really good runner (in fact, he is good at all sports, which is really annoying), told me to smile while I'm running. If you think that is easy, think again. I didn't enjoy running, but a couple of things happened when I just plastered a smile on my face. For a start, I simply couldn't tense my trapezius muscles and keep smiling. So bye bye tight neck muscles. But people would smile back at me as I ran past them — and that made my runs more enjoyable.

Studies have confirmed that smiles are contagious. Smiling also makes us look more attractive to others. It lifts our mood and the moods of those around us. This was neatly demonstrated in a Swedish study, in which people were shown pictures of a variety of emotions like joy, anger and fear. When the study subjects were looking at a picture of someone smiling, the researchers asked them to frown. But that was no easy task — they actually smiled! It turns out they had to really focus to frown — it was easier to smile back.

When you feel the weight of the world on your shoulders, walking around smiling can seem like a pipe dream. So remember again to try to fake it till you make it. I do it all the time if I'm on TV, sitting and waiting for a question or listening to another panellist or host; I keep a smile on my face as default. It keeps me relaxed and calm.

Step back a minute

My patients all know I am constantly reading and recommending self-help books. (I have an issue!) But allow me to steal a line from a really good one: *A New Earth: Awakening to your life's purpose*, by Eckhart Tolle, who also wrote *The Power of Now*. He writes: 'The primary cause of unhappiness is never the situation but your thoughts about it.' Let me see if I can expand on this magnificent concept. Sometimes it is not the situation you're in that distresses you per se, but the layers of crap you build on top of it. The example Tolle himself always refers to is being stuck in a traffic jam. If it's just a traffic jam, and you'll get wherever you're going when you get there, and meanwhile you'll listen to some awesome podcasts, then it's OK. But if your head moves on to horrific consequences of being late — 'My boss will yell at me, I will get a black mark against my name at work, I'll lose that client or I'll lose my job,' you go into a world of stress. That stress is because of the way you're thinking about it — not really the traffic jam as such.

Let's say you're diagnosed with high blood pressure. You now have three months to try to do some more exercise, drop some weight and cut back on salt or you might need to start taking medication. I often see a look of horror in a patient's eye with such a diagnosis. It's as if I can see their brains racing forwards, thinking: 'Now I am sick and I have an old person's disease and I'm going to be on tablets for the rest of my life like an old lady and have to go to the doctor all the time and the doctor said I'm fat and now I'm going to have to give up everything I like to eat and drink and live like an invalid.' I know that's an exaggeration, but exactly what is stressful? The fact that you have a diagnosis of high blood pressure, or the stuff that you have built into that story? Let's be positive: it's a good thing we picked it up now and you won't get kidney damage because you'll get awesome treatment.

In any stressful situation, try stepping back. What are the absolute irrefutable facts? And what is the negative drama you've loaded onto the facts? Get rid of the drama and free yourself.

Break it down

Sometimes the task at hand, the problem you face, is so enormous you just feel overwhelmed by the sheer weight of it all. You have to break it up into small, manageable components that you can tick off one day at a time, and put off dealing with the big picture until you're a little stronger.

I am a big list-maker. Sometimes when I feel overwhelmed by everything I have to do, I write it all down and it turns out not to be as much in reality as it *feels* in my head. (Plus there's an amazing feeling that comes from ticking stuff off my list.)

Allow time for downloading

Women spend all day uploading information like maniacs, without properly filing the clutter inside our brains. You need to allocate some time to think, if only to get the hurricane in your head sorted. I recommend you combine this with exercise, as the two go perfectly hand in hand. One thing that happens when you go on a nice long solitary walk or run or swim is that your head just zones out. All of a sudden your brain stops uploading and there's a window of opportunity — you will end up downloading, like it or not. If you don't control your downloading time, it will control you at a time when you really don't want it. Like at 3am. (Anne sounded a little strange on the phone yesterday — maybe she's upset with you for some reason? Are your children spending too long on their screens? Oh my God, you didn't pay the gas bill!) Give your brain the proper space and time to sort this stuff out.

Surround yourself with good energy

One huge study that ran for 20 years confirmed what we have suspected for a long time: being happy and content is contagious, and sad sacks gravitate towards each other. In fact, if just one of your friends is happy, it increases the likelihood that you are happy by 15 per cent! Even a friend of a friend, or the friend of a spouse or a sibling, if they are happy, it increases your chances by 10 per cent. It's obvious. Happy people are great to be around and make you enjoy yourself.

Lots of us have people in our lives whose bad energy brings us down. The phone number you dread seeing come up on your phone, the person with whom a visit is a chore. If those people are in your family, or are good friends going through a temporary hard time, you have to grin and bear it. But make your exposure as quick as possible and reward yourself by seeing a fun friend straight after to detox those negative vibes.

And then there's your home. Lots of women I speak to find their home a stress zone, rather than the harbour of tranquillity they need. Either they have lost control and have stopped trying to make sense of the chaos around them in the limited time they have available, or they see the home as the one area over which they have some control. They then spend so much time and energy making it tidy and organised that this meticulously clean and tidy home becomes a stress-generator itself.

Of all of the places in your world, you want your home to be a place of low stress. You should feel your breathing rate slow down as you walk through the door, not speed up in anxiety at the state of it! But the smallest changes can yield big results in bringing calm to your home.

Good music

Music is a perennial cultural de-stressor. If you are feeling uptight, a soft, rhythmic melody can really help bring you some inner peace. Studies have linked relaxing music with less stress in general, including lower cortisol levels. It suppresses your sympathetic nervous system that causes rapid heart rate. So you can see how switching on the Adele playlist might work for you after the day from hell at work! Similar findings have emerged from studies of people who play an instrument themselves. For me, picking up the guitar is an instant de-stressing activity (even if it means stress for those poor family members who have to listen to me play).

Green thumbs

I am such a neat freak that if I enter a house with a thousand little pots of African violets and half-watered droopy peace lilies, I start to hyperventilate. But it turns out that nice-looking, well-maintained greenery does wonders for the soul. Let's face it: in this day and age we spend more than 85 per cent of our lives indoors. Being exposed to plants in the room with you suppresses your sympathetic nervous system, so it lowers your blood pressure and also makes you feel soothed and relaxed. Could it just be cleaner air? Plant-filled rooms contain up to 60 per cent fewer airborne moulds and bacteria than plantless rooms.

Which plant? It's hard to say for sure. But there was one study inside an office building, looking at different kinds of plants with different hues of green, different smells and different sizes. The people participating in the study were measured with everything from an electroencephalogram (EEG) and electrocardiogram (ECG) to respiration rates when standing near these different plants as well as reporting on their moods. The results? Small, green, slightly scented plants scored best across the board.

Aromatherapy

Studies are a little shaky, but aromatherapists agree that scents really do help generate a sense of tranquillity. My patients are used to coming into a surgery where there's always some incense, candle, oil burner or reed diffuser.

My partners in the surgery call my room the 'day spa'. I'm a smell monster, but my smell fetish does have a tiny bit of grounding in science.

There have been a few small trials of various essential oils, either inhaled or massaged in, for mood swings. Participants in these studies reported feeling less moody and there was also a drop in their salivary-cortisol levels. The oils studied include clary sage, rosemary, lavender and bergamot, but there are practically no downsides (besides cost and the scents, which can be polarising!) so I'd go for whatever scent you like. Not because of the science, which is pretty weak, but because you enjoy it.

Get a pet

I'm biased here — I just love Freddy and Ginger, my dogs. I'm hardly surprised that 98 per cent of pet owners consider their pet to be a member of the family. Freddy and Ginger make me laugh and I love how happy they are to see me when I come home from work. To watch them run around the park is pure joy — for them and me!

Studies have more or less confirmed my personal experience that just being near a pet is good for mental and physical health. Human–animal interaction has been found to improve everything from social behaviour, interpersonal interactions and mood, to stress-related measurable parameters such as cortisol, heart rate and blood pressure. The interaction also reduces self-reported fear and anxiety and cardiovascular disease. There is also emerging evidence that interacting with animals reduces sympathetic nervous system overactivity. This improves your immune system function and ability to handle pain. It also seems to improve your level of trust towards others, reduce your aggression and improve your empathy. And it seems to do all of these things by impacting on your oxytocin levels in your brain.

In a survey of pet owners, 74 per cent said they experienced better mental health from owning a pet. And 75 per cent said that mental health benefit had extended to their friends and family members. Pet therapy has been shown to be beneficial, especially for teenagers and for the elderly.

If you live in an apartment or pet ownership is not an option for another reason, maybe get a pet fix by dog-walking at a local animal shelter, or head to the local park and play ball with someone else's dog!

Eat something

Yesterday I saw Janine, a 54-year-old educator. She came in because she'd noticed she was getting more and more anxious at the end of the day. Anxious, light-headed and even a bit nauseous. She'd snap at her students, snap at her fellow teachers and even at the parents. She was getting very busy at work; she'd been given extra classes to supervise, extra reports to write, extra junior teachers to mentor. When I quizzed her a bit it turned out she was grabbing a coffee before work at 7am and then not stopping to eat until she got home at 5pm.

'Can you see what's wrong with this picture?' I asked her. 'You're hangry!' Most of the studies of low blood sugar and its effects on mood and brainpower have been done on diabetics. But, in my experience, eating a decent lunch will help you stay calmer and less light-headed and snappy in the afternoons.

Just say no

Trying to do exactly this has been a real journey for me personally and, while I'm not sure I'll ever be 100 per cent comfortable pushing back at people, I am getting better. And I'm much happier. For me, it is all about work. It started about a year ago. At that stage, I would get in to the surgery every day about an hour before my first patient was due. I would check results, read specialist letters and action the items they requested. I would check pathology and radiology results and triage them. And then — with dread — I would open my office intramail. There were, and still often are, between 10 and 30 messages. Can I call someone who wants to talk about 'something' with me? Someone lost a blood-test form, script or referral, can I please redo it? Can I ring the mother, father, daughter to discuss? Someone needs to check something I told them in the consultation. If each call takes 5–6 minutes, 30 calls takes 150 minutes. It was getting on top of me. Wanting to 'do the right thing' for my patients meant I didn't get home to eat dinner with my family. I couldn't walk my dogs or discuss things with my husband. I couldn't pop in on my mum. I couldn't connect with friends on a weeknight because I didn't get home until 9pm. I started to resent work and resent my patients. I had even started to think about bailing out of the entire profession. And my patients are all so lovely! And I really *love* being a GP. The situation had become ridiculous.

So I just decided not to do it anymore. It's a decision I made to protect my happiness and my desire to stay in general practice. I still come in early as I did before, but the list of requests in my inbox is now a firm maybe. I chatted to my practice manager, and reprints of lost pieces of paper are done by her or our nurses. And chats are done via a consultation during allocated work hours, not by phone after hours. That has made for a much shorter list of things I feel I have to sort out. Of course, for me there might be consequences of making this firm stand: some patients might choose to see a doctor who is always available for a phone call. That's a totally reasonable decision and I fully respect it. But this change is working for me and I'm back to loving my work and my lovely patients.

You *can* say no when the cost of saying yes is your own happiness and the happiness of the people you care about most. It doesn't mean you're not nice or kind or sympathetic. It means you put a price on your own wellbeing, and that's a good thing.

MENTAL HEALTH
THE BOTTOM LINE

A whole lot of things get wrapped up into the term 'mental health'. At the most serious end of the spectrum, severe mental illness makes living a normal life close to impossible, shortens life expectancy and is potentially fatal. This deserves its own book.

In the middle we see anxiety and depression (ranging from mild to severe), which can have an impact on your life, as well as the lives of those around you. Menopause increases the risk of these conditions.

And then there is the general stress and malaise many of us feel when we hit a certain age and stage in life. Again, menopause can seem to make these stresses come to the fore.

Whatever place and space you find yourself in, put the time and effort in to maximising your mental health. Whether it's sprucing up your sleep, diet and home pot-plant life or choosing to see a psychologist with or without a medication on top, recognising the problem is the first step.

CHAPTER 6

TIRED, BLOATED AND ITCHY: THE GIRL BAND NOBODY WANTS TO SIGN

So, you've reached this time in your life when potentially you have fewer financial dramas than when you were younger, you're feeling more confident, and you're ready to enjoy a healthy middle-age. But perhaps there are some niggly, vague little symptoms just taking the edge off your enjoyment. Not the flushes anymore, thank goodness; both those and your vagina are enjoying a smooth ride thanks to the measures you've taken. But little symptoms: some tiredness, some bloating and vague tummy discomfort, and some persistent aches and pains, or maybe an unbearable all-over itch? Let's decode those symptoms and get you feeling 100 per cent.

Why am I tired all the time?

Fatigue is common across the board. We're exhausted — we all do too much — but it can take a turn for the worse around perimenopause. Are you getting enough sleep? It sounds silly but I can't tell you the number of women I see wondering whether there is 'something wrong' with them, and not connecting their chronic lack of sleep to their fatigue.

While 10–15 per cent of the population in general are chronic long-term insomniacs, sleep becomes a huge issue for many women around menopause time. Between 40 and 60 per cent of women get insomnia during perimenopause and menopause. As well as being really annoying and exhausting and making you snap at everyone around you, sleeplessness has some pretty dire consequences. Poor sleep is a risk factor for cardiovascular disease and high blood pressure, dementia, diabetes and obesity. It also weakens your immune system, increases inflammation in your body and sharpens your sensitivity to pain. Insomnia ultimately ups your risk of mental health problems such as anxiety and depression. It plays havoc with your thinking, motor skills and memory. Generally it causes frustration, worry, anger and resentment. Having insomnia can shorten your life span by eight to 10 years.

This is a terrible issue that is hardly ever acknowledged, let alone addressed properly. So why does sleep go to hell during menopause?

It's your hormones!

We're pretty sure insomnia is largely related to oestrogen deficiency leading to hot flushes. The evidence most often cited for this claim is a 2015 literature review that found taking HRT can improve chronic insomnia in menopausal women on its own without any additional therapies. With menopause comes hot flushes and, as your body temperatures soar, your sleep quality suffers.

Lower melatonin

Melatonin, made in the pineal gland that is buried deep in the brain, is the hormone that controls your circadian rhythms. Its presence in your bloodstream makes you very, very drowsy indeed. It's like an inbuilt natural sleeping pill. The suprachiasmatic nucleus (SCN), which sits in the hypothalamus, acts like a circadian pacemaker controlling your sleep–wake cycle. The SCN stimulates melatonin synthesis by the pineal gland. Being in light switches off melatonin, while darkness switches it on; turning on a light at night strongly and immediately suppresses your melatonin secretion.

Menopausal women have lower levels of melatonin; the levels drop off slowly as you approach menopause. This is partly due to natural aging, which sees the circadian system work less efficiently and decreases your melatonin secretion altogether. This happens in your mid-forties to fifties and gives you restless sleep and extra trips to the toilet at night. Melatonin levels are also smashed by fibromyalgia, depression, sleep apnoea and chronic obstructive pulmonary disease (also called emphysema).

Higher orexin
Discovered in 1998, orexins are chemicals found throughout the brain that contribute to wakefulness. In fact, without orexins we'd all suffer from narcolepsy and not be able to stay awake. Because orexins are so recent in terms of discovery, we're slowly unpacking everything they do. But higher orexin A levels have been linked in studies to higher blood-sugar levels, a worse pattern of high cholesterol, higher blood pressure and higher body mass index.

It seems that menopause causes higher blood levels of orexin A. Interestingly, HRT lowers orexin A so might help sleep that way. You can get orexin receptor blockers, called Suvorexant, on prescription from your doctor. In some studies, Suvorexant increased 'sleep efficiency' and the amount of sleep by 22–50 minutes a night. Sadly, the other studies that have been done haven't been as amazing. On the plus side, Suvorexant doesn't appear to be addictive.

Disrupted cortisol
Cortisol normally has a fairly predictable peak and trough cycle over 24 hours. Before menopause, we have very low or even undetectable cortisol levels around midnight that build up overnight to peak first thing in the morning. Cortisol levels then decline slowly over the course of the day. Around the time of menopause, studies have shown higher cortisol levels through the night than the usual morning cortisol spike. Oestrogen helps regulate the cortisol cycle back to early morning peak and night-time sleep. Unfortunately, sleep deprivation causes high cortisol levels, which inhibits a decent sleep. This can be a real vicious cycle.

How can I fix my sleep?

I'm going to discuss medications last and start with the simple things you can do without even entering a doctor's surgery.

Overhaul your sleep hygiene

I'm not talking about your dirty sheets here — I'm talking about rotten sleep habits. No matter what else we do to try to wrangle your sleep back into gear, sleep hygiene will always be on the list of strategies.

Over years, or even decades, bad sleepers have often developed bad habits that unconsciously program their brains not to sleep. The idea of sleep hygiene is to clean up those bad sleep habits and retrain the brain to know when it's sleep time and when it's not. Here are the most important sleep hygiene steps to rewire your brain.

You need a wind-down period before bed. This is a good hour or so to allow your overstimulated brain to calm down, with no screens of any kind, be they TV, iPad, iPhone or whatever. The blue light from screens that hits the retina at the back of the eyes inhibits melatonin release from your brain and stops you both falling and staying asleep. Ideally we should get off screens for an hour before bedtime; meanwhile, in the real world, that's close to impossible. So for less than $10 you can buy glasses in orange that promise to filter out blue light and allow your brain to make more melatonin. Studies are pretty thin on the ground but these are a low-cost punt and anecdotally many people have found some benefit. Meanwhile, you can activate the blue light filter on your phone from around 8pm.

Also, no heart-stopping books or arguments before bed. Instead, try soft music, an aromatherapy bath, dim lights and maybe a nice orgasm if you have a partner who is willing and able!

The next step is to try to get to bed at around the same time each night. The idea here is to switch your body clock back on and get your body used to associating sleep with a certain time.

Step three is to train your brain to wake up at roughly the same time every day (give or take 30 minutes). Barring an all-nighter with Mum who's been taken to hospital, or a teenager who comes home from a party at 4am, or other exceptional circumstances, your brain needs to learn to wake up in the morning, shut down pineal melatonin production and feel bright and awake during the daytime. This routine includes weekends. Not forever, but just until we sort out your brain and get you sleeping well again. And no daytime naps: short-term gain for night-time pain!

Your bed is for sex and sleep only. There is a fallacy that 'just resting' in bed is good for your brain. But it actually has the opposite effect, making it harder for your brain to fall asleep later on.

Once you get into bed (or have finished having sex), practise progressive muscular relaxation — relax your muscles one by one from the tips of your toes to the top of your head. (See also the mindfulness meditation in Chapter 5). There is some evidence for yoga and abdominal breathing, too.

Give yourself 15 minutes to fall asleep. If in that time your mind starts to wander or you feel tense, get up and leave the room for somewhere between 10 and 30 minutes and then return to bed as if you were starting the night again. It doesn't matter what you do as long as you don't over-stimulate your brain with a screen! You could even get some ironing done. If you're awake anyway, at least you'll achieve some productive work and not feel quite as frustrated as you do when you're just lying and watching the clock for hours.

Avoid large meals and limit fluid intake in the evenings. Big meals increase your risk of having gastro-oesophageal reflux (feeling uncomfortable in the guts) and drinking too much will guarantee multiple trips to the loo.

Check your bedroom environment

It seems pretty basic, but is your bedroom a sleep-friendly place? For example, light is a sleep killer because it stops melatonin kicking in. If you have issues with sheer curtains, bright street lights or the hall light outside your door, you might find it interferes with your sleep. Try rearranging your bedroom furniture to face away from the light, or wear an eye mask.

How old is your mattress? The mattress companies tell you to change them over every 10 years. I'm innately sceptical about these promotions but an unsponsored study out of the US found that indeed changing the mattress improved sleep quality and reduced back pain.

Not only do old mattresses give you uncomfortable human-shaped divots to roll into and get stuck in, but they are often full of mould and dust-mite faeces that can give your allergies a work-out if you have hay fever. And the ideal mattress for the best sleep? It is not an area science has embraced, but 75 per cent of orthopaedic surgeons recommend firm or hard mattresses for the relief of back pain. Mattress technology 'toppers' now help regulate temperature (see Chapter 3, Baptism by fire).

Exercise

This is generally recommended for people who are having difficulty sleeping. In some studies, people with insomnia seem to fall asleep more quickly, sleep slightly longer and report a better night's sleep after four to 24 weeks of exercising than before they started their work-outs.

Researchers don't really know why this happens. Possibly because you cool down after exercise; possibly because it helps manage anxiety. Regardless, exercise is a good thing to do for almost every condition linked to menopause.

Yoga

A randomised, parallel group study conducted over a six-month period compared an hour of yoga six days a week, with Ayurvedic therapy, and something called 'no therapy at all' in 69 older adults.

The yogis experienced a one-hour increase in their total sleep time, compared to before they started the yoga. That was far superior to the zero help or Ayurveda groups. That pretty much reflects other studies of yoga and sleep.

Tai chi

Tai chi is a low- to moderate-intensity Chinese exercise that includes a meditation component. A study of the effects of tai chi (consisting of three 60-minute sessions a week for 24 weeks) in 118 older adults in comparison to low-impact exercise noted that tai chi improved self-reported sleep duration by 48 minutes. General health-related quality of life and daytime sleepiness levels also improved. No injuries were reported in either group.

Of note, 33 per cent of subjects withdrew from the study (with no significant difference between the tai chi and exercise groups). If these findings are replicated by additional research using objective measures, tai chi could add to the range of complementary and alternative medicine treatment options available for insomnia.

Ditch the (excess) alcohol

Any more than one glass of wine and I get really drowsy. But that doesn't mean alcohol helps me sleep well. Quite the opposite: it stuffs up the quality of our sleep. Specifically, it blocks REM sleep, which is restorative sleep, so we often wake feeling groggy. Excuse the pun.

There are a few reasons for the disruption. The volume of liquid can make you need to pee through the night; it can make oesophageal reflux worse, which can wake you from heartburn; and it can make sleep-disordered breathing or sleep apnoea worse (see page 159). Stick to one or two drinks a night.

I still can't sleep. What about medications?

HRT

Studies have found some pretty interesting answers to whether HRT will improve your sleep around menopause. It turns out HRT improves sleep quality in women with hot flushes, but if there are no flushes it is somewhat less effective. Combining HRT with sleep hygiene, relaxation techniques and the like has been shown in studies to be more effective than HRT alone.

Antihistamines

There are some medications that have sleepiness as a side effect. Diphenhydramine and doxylamine are over-the-counter 'first-generation' antihistamines that have sedation as a side effect. They're also the main ingredients in a lot of over-the-counter sleeping tablets you can get at the pharmacy. They last in your body for around nine hours, so many people feel a bit drunk the next morning. In my experience they work well with no addiction. They are best for Friday nights or a time when an antihistamine hangover won't ruin your day.

Low-dose antidepressants

There is one called Mirtazapine that has sedation as a side effect. You need a prescription from your GP for this but currently it is not approved as a sleeping pill, only as an antidepressant. There are a couple of problems with this; firstly, it is approved for use as an antidepressant only, so you need to understand you would be using it for a condition for which it isn't approved. Also, it can make you very hungry, so long-term weight gain can be a problem. That puts many of my patients off!

Amitriptyline is another, older antidepressant often used by GPs for insomnia. It is generally used in this way at very low doses (far lower than the dose for depression) but we don't have good data on the costs and benefits of this.

Benzodiazepine sleeping pills

These are your classic 'tranquillisers'. They work by activating the GABA receptors in the brain, mimicking the GABA relaxation and sleeping hormone. I prescribe them short-term for insomnia during a crisis. I've had patients who lose their job or find out their partner has cancer and cannot sleep a wink. They are not a long-term solution and can be used for a maximum of two weeks before you start running into issues with addiction. They can cause drowsiness the next day and make you more likely to trip and fall over if you wake up in the middle of the night for a visit to the loo. So they're not a solution for menopausal insomnia.

Non-benzodiazepine sleeping pills

The big one here is Suvorexant, the new orexin antagonist. As we already discussed, it's relatively new but looks effective and without the addiction levels we see in benzodiazepines. We don't recommend taking it for more than three months because we don't have studies for longer than that. I'd still prefer to see all medications as an emergency measure, rather than as a long-term option for menopausal insomnia.

Melatonin supplements

You can get melatonin tablets on prescription from your doctor. In Australia they're only advocated strongly for people over the age of 65 but studies have shown them to be effective for women in perimenopause and post-menopause well before the age of 65. The best thing about using melatonin is that it isn't addictive and doesn't give you a hangover in the morning. As a medication, it has a relatively mild hypnotic effect as compared to other sleeping pills.

And what about complementary therapies and home remedies?

I love a good statistic and this one staggered me: a recent analysis of the National Health Interview Survey (NHIS) in the US found that while 4.5 per cent of adults had used some form of complementary medicine for their insomnia in the past year, up to 10 per cent of the same group in the survey had used a prescription sedative. Seriously? Having read about the options your GP can give you in the prescription space, why would anyone take a sleeping pill? Because sleep deprivation is so bad! I know. Anyway, let's go through some other complementary, alternative and home remedy options together.

Aromatherapy

This is a general practice of inhaling essential oils, with the aim of the scents having calming and hypnotic effects on the brain. It can be practised in a few ways:

◆ Direct application of essential oils to your skin. That's going to be pretty strong, so it can be diluted with a carrier oil such as sweet almond oil. You can dab the oil onto your temples, forehead and wrists before bedtime.

◆ Apply a few drops of essential oil onto a cotton ball and slip it inside your pillowcase at night.

◆ Before sleep, take a bath with a few drops of essential oil added to the water.

- Add essential oil drops to a humidifier or vaporiser in the bedroom at bedtime.
- Just sniff directly from the bottle of essential oil before going to sleep.
- Add a few drops of essential oil to a warm, damp cloth and put this over your forehead or neck.
- Fill a spray bottle with water and a few drops of essential oil, then spray the mixture over your pillowcase and bedsheets before sleep.

The evidence for essential oils for insomnia tends to come from small trials that aren't great quality. The best evidence exists for lavender, chamomile, ylang ylang, jasmine, bergamot and sweet marjoram.

I don't think anyone would say these are the be-all-and-end-all of insomnia cures, but added to other treatments, they will not hurt and might help a lot. Some people have very sensitive skin and can get rashes if they come in direct contact with some essential oils. So, skin-patch test first.

Valerian

Derived from the *Valeriana officinalis* plant, valerian attaches to both the GABA and serotonin receptors in the brain and makes you sleepier and a bit cheerier. There have been a few studies of valerian and many of those were randomised, placebo-controlled trials. From those trials you could say there is some evidence of improvement in sleep with valerian, if you take it for two weeks or more, at least on subjective testing. Objective testing, however, shows little to no improvement in sleep. Valerian was combined with lemon balm specifically for menopausal women in one placebo-controlled trial of 100 women. It had some reasonable results and there are few side effects. I'd give it a shot.

Acupuncture

There are small, poor-quality trials, but they're hard to draw any firm conclusions from. A review of 12 tiny studies of acupuncture for insomnia in postmenopausal women with or without hot flushes found 'overall positive effects'. And yet the authors gave it a firm 'maybe'. That's because the studies were pretty poor, giving insufficient hardcore evidence to support acupuncture for insomnia. So, bottom line, it's a firm no for hot flushes and a firm maybe for insomnia.

Meditation

See page 124 for a guide to mediating. This has been specifically studied as a treatment for insomnia. Randomised controlled studies of various meditation techniques have been shown to help you fall asleep more quickly and stay asleep longer. And these results are seen using both patient reports and quantitative measures of sleep. A small study of 30 women who had insomnia postmenopause found that an eight-week mindfulness meditation course helped with sleep quality, quality of life, attention levels and even fewer hot flushes!

Magnesium supplements

As I mentioned in Chapter 5, magnesium is a mineral found in fibre-rich foods. Think dark green veggies, such as kale, along with legumes, such as kidney beans, nuts and whole grains. No wonder that, at least in the US, studies consistently show that our intake of magnesium is inadequate.

Some evidence shows that magnesium supplements can help you get off to sleep. Small studies have found that magnesium supplements may help older people fall asleep quicker. It seems to also help people with restless leg syndrome. It might be because it appears to increase the amount of the neurotransmitter GABA in the brain. This can effectively slow your head down, allowing your brain to switch off and fall asleep.

You can't overdose on magnesium in foods, but you *can* take too many supplements, especially if they're bound to a chemical that can upset your guts. Forms of magnesium, such as magnesium carbonate, chloride and oxide, can all cause stomach cramps and diarrhoea. It's better to use magnesium glycinate or magnesium gluconate.

Might I have sleep apnoea?

Do you snore? Loudly? Do you snore and sometimes stop breathing altogether? This can be hard to pick up when you live alone, or when your partner sleeps like a log and doesn't pay attention to your snoring at night. These are all signs of sleep apnoea. If the answer to your snoring is unknown but you wake up exhausted every day and then easily nod off at the drop of a hat, those are also signs that you might have sleep apnoea. As are waking to pee in the night and also waking with a headache and a dry mouth.

Sleep apnoea happens when your breathing reduces substantially at night while you're asleep so your oxygen levels drop, including the oxygen to your brain. There are two basic types: obstructive sleep apnoea and central sleep apnoea. Most common is obstructive sleep apnoea, in which the upper airway becomes blocked repeatedly during sleep, so it either partially or even completely stops airflow. Central sleep apnoea is rarer and involves the brain not sending signals to the airways to tell them to breathe. Prior to menopause, women are only a third as likely as men to have sleep apnoea. That changes after menopause when the numbers even out.

To diagnose sleep apnoea I often order a sleep study, to be done either at home or in a specialised lab. The study allows the specialist to record the number of episodes of slow or stopped breathing in an hour, and also diagnose the extent of low oxygen levels in the blood during episodes of 'apnoea'.

Obstructive sleep apnoea is more common if you have a lot of tissue around your neck area. And by 'tissue' I mean fat — and big muscles. Accumulating fat around the neck is a big risk — and, while it can happen at any age, the older you are, the more common it is. Higher alcohol consumption also increases your risk, possibly because it relaxes the muscles around the airways, making them more likely to collapse. Other risk factors include smoking and being overweight or obese. There is also a genetic link.

Not only does it leave you feeling tired most of the time, but sleep apnoea can also be linked to some pretty disabling symptoms and conditions, so it is important to treat. It seems that sleep apnoea increases inflammation in your body generally. This might be why it increases your risk of:

- Asthma
- Atrial fibrillation (a funny heart rhythm linked to strokes)

- Cancers, including pancreatic, kidney and skin cancers

- Chronic kidney disease

- Dementia in older adults

- Heart attacks, heart failure, difficult-to-control high blood pressure and strokes

- Eye problems such as glaucoma and dry eye

- Pre-diabetes, insulin resistance and type 2 diabetes

Apart from addressing risk factors by getting you to lose weight, give up smoking and cut down on alcohol, we do have specific treatments for sleep apnoea. Breathing devices such as continuous positive air pressure (CPAP) machines are effective at not only improving your sleep quality and making you feel more awake during the day, but also reducing your risk of those associated diseases.

Could it be a thyroid problem that's making me tired?

I always keep thyroid disease in the back of my mind for women, especially around menopause time. Thyroid disease is predominantly a women's problem: women are between five and 20 times more likely to get a thyroid problem than men. About 7.6 per cent of women have an underactive thyroid gland at any time, but that number rises to 17 per cent in women over 70 years of age. When you consider that the chance of thyroid disease increases with age, around menopause it should be on your doctor's radar. And thyroid disease will leave you feeling exhausted.

The thyroid gland, located in the neck just below the throat, produces your two main thyroid hormones: tetraiodothyronine (thyroxine, T4) and triiodothyronine (T3). These hormones act on cells in organs with a wide range of effects. Thyroid hormones regulate protein, carbohydrate and fat metabolism. T3 is the most active form, while T4 has only minimal hormonal activity but travels around the body turning into T3 wherever it is needed.

Many of my patients diagnosed with a thyroid problem want to know why it has happened. We usually don't know. The most common cause of an underactive thyroid is an immune system problem, such as Hashimoto thyroiditis, when your immune system attacks your own thyroid for reasons we don't quite understand. The other big cause is doctors! Our use of radiotherapy for head and neck cancers, as well as medications such as Lithium, Amiodarone, Interferon and some types of chemotherapy for cancer, can all cause subsequent thyroid problems. Our use of radioiodine or surgery for benign or malignant thyroid diseases can also contribute to subsequent thyroid problems.

Diagnosing your thyroid problem might be difficult because many of the symptoms, such as anxiety, heart palpitations, sweating, hot flushes, gaining weight and insomnia, are common for both the thyroid and menopause. So just keep it in mind.

Apart from the obvious (making you feel better), there is a huge imperative to treat thyroid disease. Unrecognised, untreated thyroid problems can give you an increased risk of cardiovascular disease, bone fractures, cognitive impairment (and maybe dementia), depression and earlier death.

So, how do you fix thyroid disease? For an overactive thyroid we might wait, as often it will become underactive with time, or treat it with medication or even iodine therapy. The best treatment for an underactive gland (which is more common than overactive) is the replacement of the missing hormone by taking a simple tablet every day. In most cases, we only replace the thyroxine (T4) and trust that your body will break that down to get adequate amounts of the T3 it needs. Very rarely do we need to give you T3, but it is available.

Getting the hormone level right can take a few weeks or months, but thyroid hormone therapy fixes the problem with close to no side effects. Lots of my patients expect to feel better the next day but it takes a couple of weeks for the fatigue to improve, and then six to eight weeks for blood levels of thyroid hormone to stabilise. You need a prescription and your doctor will monitor your TSH levels to confirm you're on the right dose. Thyroid hormone tablets can be annoying to take because they need to be kept cool — preferably in a fridge — making travel difficult.

Your diet matters when you start thyroid replacement therapy. The following can all make thyroid hormone tablets less effective:

- Walnuts
- Soybean flour
- Iron supplements or multivitamins containing iron
- Calcium supplements
- Antacids
- Some medications (check with your pharmacist)

As you get older, your doctor will need to make adjustments to your thyroid replacement medication. Sometimes we have to lower the dose because you start metabolising and clearing the drugs in your system more slowly. You might realise your dose is too high because you feel hot or develop palpitations. Or we might pick it up with a routine blood test.

It's common to need *more* thyroid replacement hormone to keep your thyroid levels in balance as you age. This is because thyroid function naturally declines over time. Once again, you might notice you feel tired or feel the cold and think immediately of your thyroid. Alternatively, a blood test might pick it up. It does go to show the importance of monitoring your thyroid hormone levels, especially when you're on medication.

Might my iron be too low?

Iron is the molecule at the centre of haemoglobin, the chemical in red blood cells that transports oxygen from lungs to tissues where it is used as fuel. Lack of iron is one of the biggest causes of exhaustion and even a bit of depression. And the number-one cause of iron deficiency in women of any age, but especially leading into menopause, is *heavy, heavy* periods. And now we have hit on one of the most common hormonal problems I see in women in perimenopause; it's not something women talk about, even to their doctor. We tend to expect to bleed heavily at the age when menopause is approaching and we just don't discuss it. But heavy periods can wreak havoc with your body.

Between 9 and 20 per cent of women run around with an iron deficiency–anaemia issue. I can't tell you how many of my women patients — at both ends of the menstrual era: youngish teens or late forties — come in with some general complaint that smacks of an iron issue. Sure enough, when I run blood tests, they reveal shocking iron deficiency. And when I ask the question about periods I hear sorry tales of heavy bleeding, overflowing, clots and exhaustion.

If you are low in iron you will probably feel exhausted and weak, you will have a dodgy immune system and catch more little infections. You might feel the cold and feel light-headed. In more severe cases you might experience a rapid heartbeat, leg cramps and shortness of breath when you exercise. In my experience, women with iron deficiency also get more headaches and migraines. And, a weird one, you might even crave ice! And then the periods themselves . . . not all women recognise that their periods are heavy.

So what's a normal period?

A normal menstrual cycle is 21–35 days per cycle, and normal bleeding lasts an average of seven days with a flow of between 10 and 60ml in total over those seven days. Over 80ml earns you the diagnosis of menorrhagia (heavy periods). I don't expect you to measure your flow (although these days, with the enormous popularity of moon cups, more women do). We can usually tell just by chatting to you. And I always ask about blood clots. Clots are not normal in a period and tell me that your flow is too heavy. Periods lasting a week or more are not normal. Ditto having to wake up during the night to change a pad or tampon; even just once during a period.

Heavy periods are ridiculously common and can make perimenopause a living hell. Around one in five women faces an issue at this time. Researchers at the University of Michigan went into this in a bit of depth. They found that 91 per cent of perimenopausal women had had periods lasting ten or more days between once and three times in the previous three years. Nearly

88 per cent said they'd had six or more days of spotting, and almost 78 per cent had three or more days of heavy flow. And more than a quarter of the women had as many as three periods in the previous six months that had lasted more than ten days.

It's not about the volume of blood per se, but the effects of the heavy bleeding. In my experience, heavy periods can make you avoid exercise, avoid sex, interrupt your sleep and be *very* expensive (pads and tampons cost way too much). And the amount of blood you lose can make you feel exhausted from iron deficiency. So, let's look at the causes of heavy bleeding.

Anovulation (not ovulating)

As you hit perimenopause, your hypothalamus and pituitary are working pretty normally, but your ovaries don't perform as well. The follicle-stimulating hormone (FSH) doesn't get those tired old follicles to develop as well, resulting in lacklustre production of oestrogen. There's enough oestrogen around to get a nice thick lining of the uterus (endometrium), but the suboptimal follicles do not respond to an luteinising hormone (LH) surge; as a result they do not ovulate and you don't get a corpus luteum. No corpus luteum means no progesterone. No progesterone means no maturation of the endometrium. This state is what we call 'unopposed oestrogen'. You get a thick overblown endometrium but it's disorganised. When it finally outgrows its blood supply and degenerates, there is chaotic breakdown of the endometrial lining at different levels. That is why 'anovulatory' bleeding is heavier than normal periods. And it can feel as if life is just one long period. You can forget the whole five days on, 23 days off business — your periods can start lasting two weeks at a time!

But, given that no two cycles are the same during perimenopause, the following month might be a pretty OK period. Either you had a low oestrogen month, or your body randomly made a pretty awesome corpus luteum and pumped out enough progesterone to counterbalance the oestrogen.

If this sounds like you, I can't tell you how long it will take. See your GP first, to rule out any other cause of the heavy bleeding and to get your iron levels measured. You can't continue to gush blood and not run out of iron at some point.

What are the options for treating my very heavy periods?

Progesterone-only treatments

I'm going to start with the absolute best treatment. I know it's your choice but pretty much every peak gynaecological body agrees: progesterone-containing IUDs are the bees' knees!

This type of IUD slows down menstrual blood loss by as much as 96 per cent. I love this little device (which I'm not legally allowed to name) because it is such an effective contraception. For women without heavy bleeding, it slows your periods down so much that you might just need a panty liner for three days. For women with menorrhagia, instead of needing double–super-maxi-reinforced tampons every hour for 10 days, you should have what you remember as a normal or even light period. Which is great for your iron stores. Get it inserted (by your GP, a women's health nurse or gynaecologist) and you won't have to think about it for five years. Initially you can have a bit of spotting for a couple of months until it settles in, but I always advise my patients to persist because it's worth it.

While I love this device, it does polarise opinion. In theory, because the progesterone is delivered directly to the lining of the uterus, not the body as a whole, side effects such as bloating, breast tenderness and mood changes are minimal. Look at enough message boards and Facebook groups and you'd think otherwise: women do tend to blame it for absolutely everything. Science dismisses this, but, in my opinion, if you feel worse on this type of IUD, then get it removed.

If you don't like the idea of sticking progesterone directly into your uterus, you can try taking it orally. In theory, these progestogens basically balance out the oestrogen in the endometrium, stopping the endometrium from overgrowing and making it more organised and packed down. You take tablets several times a day from days five to 26 of your menstrual cycle, counting the first day of your period as day one. While 20 per cent of women shut down their periods altogether with this method, for others it can cause very irregular cycles and spotting. Plus, it's not contraceptive, so we keep it in reserve for women who can't have a progesterone-containing

IUD fitted, can't take a non-hormonal treatment, such as tranexamic acid (see below), and can't take the pill. It's a last resort, really.

Even more last resort are progesterone injections into the arm every 12 weeks. Fifty per cent of women who have these stop their periods altogether. But the side effects are often unacceptable to women and their doctors alike; they include weight gain, greasy skin and hair, acne and bloating. Plus, in shutting down the natural cycle and your own oestrogen, you can get early osteoporosis. I only have one patient on this particular treatment, but she absolutely loves it. She insists it is the best thing she has ever used, and at 45 she finds it more acceptable than a progesterone-containing IUD or the pill. She knows the risks and she's OK with them.

Combined oestrogen and progesterone treatments

Going on the pill to thin the endometrium is a popular route to take. The advantages of the pill include its contraceptive effect, as well as regulating the blood flow. I always encourage continuous dosing (so, skipping your sugar pills rather than having that cyclical 'period'). This gives you much less bleeding, both in duration and amount. But you can get breakthrough bleeding and spotting, which can be annoying.

Non-hormonal treatments

A pro-clotting drug called tranexamic acid is very effective at reducing heavy bleeding. It reduces the amount of blood lost by 40 to 65 per cent and, after three months, it improves quality of life for 80 per cent of women who use it. Tablets are taken for five days during your period and, because of the (at least theoretical) increased clotting risk, you can't take it if you're on the pill. You also can't take it if you have a rare clotting disorder or some rare cardiovascular conditions. By the way, in studies, we don't see a big increase in clots.

Your GP might also try a non-steroidal anti-inflammatory drug, such as Diclofenac, mefenamic acid or Naproxen. Studies show that they can slow down heavy menstrual blood flow but are not as effective as tranexamic acid — although they can be taken together. In studies, 52 per cent of women treated with mefenamic acid for two months still lost 80ml of blood per cycle.

Non-steroidal anti-inflammatories are great if you get period pains, too. Ideally, if your cycle is regular, you'd start taking them one to two days before your period is due (depending on how severe the bleeding and pain are) and stop on day two or three of your period, depending on when your flow slows down. Side effects include stomach upset, so always take them with food.

Surgical solutions

Surgery is your last resort. Bizarrely, I find many gynaecologists still suggest a procedure called 'dilatation and curettage' (also referred to as a D&C). It's really best for getting a diagnosis. The gynaecologist sends off a sample of the endometrium to the lab to make sure there's no endometrial hyperplasia cancer or adenomyosis (see page 171). D&C is a pretty hopeless treatment because it typically works for one or two months at most. Ideally, it isn't done on its own but is combined with a progesterone-containing IUD insertion.

Alternatively, your gynaecologist might suggest something called an endometrial ablation, in which they use heated elements, liquid nitrogen, high-frequency sound waves or laser to destroy the endometrium. The advantages are firstly that it is pretty effective. Between 67 and 93 per cent of women have their flow reduced to a 'normal period' (10–60ml in total). Most women are pretty happy with the results. And it is pretty easy — endometrial ablation is generally done as a day procedure, with most women returning to work the next day. While it is really effective, all surgery comes with the risks of the anaesthetic, a significant cost and some inherent risks in the procedure, no matter how rare. That's why we doctors always chose surgery last.

The downside is that it doesn't always work and there are potential side effects. You'd have to be seriously unlucky to get pregnant after ablation, but it *can* happen. If it does, the risk of serious complications makes progressing with the pregnancy extremely difficult. So you would only have ablation if you agreed to use birth control until you're on the other side of menopause.

Hysterectomy is another surgical option, but it is only used if there is something else going on so I'll discuss it later in this chapter.

Why else might I be bleeding?

Fibroids (leiomyomas)

Around one in five women has at least one uterine fibroid during her fertile years but that booms by the age of 50, when around 80 per cent of us have them! Fibroids are benign tumours in the muscle of the uterus and, although you can get one at a time, they tend to be clustered. We don't know what causes them, except that they are hormonal and tend to be fuelled by oestrogen, so when you pass through menopause they either stop growing or shrink. We know some things increase your chances of getting fibroids, such as starting your periods early, high blood pressure, a positive family history and soy milk consumption. Being on the pill or the injectable progestogen, smoking (no, that's not a typo!), low body mass index and having had more babies reduce the risk. But, once you have fibroids and they're making you bleed, the bleeding is unlikely to stop until you get them sorted or reach full-blown menopause. Most women opt for treatment because, apart from feeling drained all the time due to a lack of iron, the constant bleeding is a pain in the neck.

Fibroids can be so tiny that you need a microscope to see them (in which case, you will never be worried by them) or they can be enormous — up to a kilogram in weight. Only half of the women with them ever get symptoms. When they do cause symptoms, as well as heavy irregular periods they can cause pressure on the bladder, chronic pelvic pain and painful sexual intercourse. In an international study of over 20,000 women, 53.7 per cent said symptoms had a negative impact on their life in the last 12 months, with the main impacts being on their sexual life (42.9 per cent), performance at work (27.7 per cent) and relationship and family (27.2 per cent).

Fibroids are often detected by symptom or incidentally but they are diagnosed by ultrasound scan, and treatment often depends on whether you've finished having babies. If you want to leave that door open, the first line of treatment is often the same progesterone-containing IUD we use for anovulatory bleeding. The tiny amount of progestin it releases stabilises the lining of the uterus and often — but not always — sorts out the bleeding.

The alternatives are basically all surgical. These include getting the artery that feeds the fibroid injected with a substance that cuts off its blood supply, making it shrink (arterial embolisation). This is brilliant if you're young, don't want a hysterectomy and have finished having a family. So you get to keep your uterus, but nix those fibroids that are contributing to heavy bleeding. You need a highly qualified specialist in the field and it's not cheap.

Surgically removing individual fibroids can be a simple op but it does depend on where they're located. If you have lots of big ones, it is more difficult technically. So if you no longer need a uterus for child-bearing, and removing the fibroids is looking tricky, you might be offered a hysterectomy. Fibroids are the leading cause for women to have hysterectomies and account for 39 per cent of all hysterectomies performed annually in the US.

Endometrial polyps

These are basically (usually) benign overgrowths of the endometrial cells that form a little growth that projects into the cavity of the uterus. They're not uncommon; in fact, they're found on ultrasound in 20 to 40 per cent of women with heavy periods. They can be tiny — around 1mm in diameter — to about the size of a golf ball or occasionally even bigger, and they hang off a thin stalk from the endometrium. Exactly like fibroids, we just don't know why they happen, but they're more common in women with high blood pressure, obesity and in women taking Tamoxifen for the treatment or prevention of breast cancer. Polyps cause heavy bleeding as they grow because they dangle from their stalks and rub on and irritate the endometrium they touch, which ultimately rubs off the endometrium and exposes the little blood vessels underneath. As with fibroids, they often shrink after menopause and, like fibroids, they tend to crop up in your forties — around the end of your fertile life. Like fibroids, unless they're visible on the cervix (I will sometimes see them when I'm doing a pap smear) they tend to be found by ultrasound scan when we're looking for the cause of irregular or heavy bleeding, or bleeding after sex.

They don't always need treatment. Up to a quarter of polyps regress or even disappear, particularly if they're less than 10mm in size. But there is a caveat: if they're causing nasty bleeding, they should be removed. If they occur after menopause, they need to be removed because — it's rare — they can be malignant. Removal does require a general anaesthetic and surgery but it can be done through the opening of the cervix without leaving any abdominal scars.

Adenomyosis

This is a wacky disease in which endometrial cells start growing into the wall of the uterus. It's a cousin of endometriosis, in which endometrial cells start growing out of the uterus altogether, on the ovaries, tubes, bowel . . . In theory, one doesn't necessarily go with the other, but Sydney gynaecologist Dr David Rosen, who is Director of the Sydney Women's Endosurgery Centre, says if you are operating on adenomyosis, there is almost always endometriosis there.

Like fibroids and polyps, this is a problem of the late forties just before menopause (unless you're unlucky and it happens earlier); it causes heavy and painful periods and often painful sex, too. The endometrium sloughs off during the period but the blood is trapped inside the uterine wall and causes the signature pain.

And, once again, we don't know what causes it. You can only properly diagnose adenomyosis by looking at the uterus tissue under a microscope, which means removing the uterus by hysterectomy. However, as ultrasounds have got better, we're diagnosing it more and more in that way — it needs an 'expert eye', such as a women's health radiologist.

I am obsessed with this condition; mostly because I diagnose it in so many patients on ultrasound, but also because I have it! So do 20 to 35 per cent of women, so we're not that unusual. I'll share my journey and what I'm doing about it, alongside the textbook version. (Will you be surprised that they don't totally align?)

This is how it all happened for me. I had a progesterone-containing IUD put in by my obstetrician at my six-week check after my last child. I *love* my IUD and I haven't had a proper period for over 20 years. Not until I hit about 48. First I started getting periods again; I had to plunder the girls' tampon stash and reintroduce myself for the first time since I was 27. And the period pain! I never had period pain, even as a teenager. The first time it happened, I thought I was dying! (My medical degree doesn't inoculate me against being a drama queen.) My GP sent me for an ultrasound scan and there it was. I have never had any symptoms of endometriosis; just the adenomyosis.

This is what I do . . . the special IUD means I have a normal or even light period (less than 60ml total blood loss) so I now once again have tampons in the bathroom at all times. And because I have a regular cycle, I start on Naproxen in the lead-up to my period and don't get too much pain.

And this is the textbook advice . . . Nobody bloody well knows what they're doing. No peak body has guidelines. It's a guidance-free zone. The progesterone-containing IUD is proposed as a treatment for the heavy bleeding (yeah, sometimes . . . I have patients for whom it simply doesn't work). And, as for pain — well, no! It doesn't work. Anti-inflammatories are suggested as a possibility (they work for me). Aromatase inhibitors (AIs) and selective estrogen receptor modulators (SERMs) have been studied for this. Horrible! They're great treatments for breast cancer but can give you horrendous hot flushes and increase your risk of blood clots. So I'm not buying.

Hysterectomy — the cure? If that makes you freak out, keep reading.

Tell me about hysterectomy then!

Seen as the barbaric butchery of women, removing the uterus is almost taboo nowadays. If I drop the H bomb on my patients, a goodly number will run screaming from the room. Many of us have been told dark family folklore that Grandma was never the same after her hysterectomy. Some doctor (no doubt, male) hacked out the heart of her femininity and she never recovered. She will have had a massive scar and every single female organ — uterus, fallopian tubes and ovaries — was removed, often throwing her into a sudden menopause, *far* more horrible than the natural menopause. These days it is usually done via keyhole surgery; only the uterus and tubes are taken, and the ovaries remain.

I am not so anti-hysterectomy. Sure, it's surgery. Sure, it needs a general anaesthetic. Sure, that is not free of risk. But:

- It will completely relieve for good whatever nasty bleeding or pain you're having.

- If you need HRT, you can have oestrogen-only HRT and be on it for longer.

- No more cervical screening tests. No cervix means no pap tests. It's a minor thing, but a little plus in life.

- Probably a lower risk of ovarian cancer — for all hysterectomy patients. Yes, we leave your ovaries in but the surgery seems to protect them. The fallopian tubes are removed with the uterus and this seems to reduce the risk of subsequent ovarian cancer.

- No cervical or uterine cancer. If you haven't got a cervix or uterus, you can't get cancer in them. (Having said that, if you've been monitored for HPV of the cervix or an abnormal pap test, you need to continue to have a vault smear, which is like a pap test except we only sample the vagina cells not the cervix.)

- You can get your stress incontinence fixed at the same time. It's a pretty easy bolt-on procedure using a couple of extra sutures.

Three myths about hysterectomy

1. You're out of action for six weeks. Reality: my patients generally stay in hospital for one to three nights (average is two). They're back to driving a week later, back to work in around three weeks and feeling back to normal after four weeks.

2. You become menopausal and grouchy. Reality: generally the ovaries are left inside, so you will get whatever oestrogen they're producing. But, for most women, menopause is nigh anyway, which is why they're having issues with that part of the anatomy in the first place.

3. Prolapse. Reality: The link between hysterectomy and prolapse is not so much a myth as a bit of an outdated fact. In the old days of straightforward abdominal hysterectomy, or even vaginal hysterectomy (when the gynaecologist removed the uterus via the vagina instead of through the tummy wall), the gynaecologist had to slice through a critical part of the pelvic floor, the 'utero-sacral ligaments', to get the

uterus out. A higher risk of prolapse was a problem with hysterectomy, although it didn't happen until around 20 years after the operation. These days, with laparoscopic hysterectomy (keyhole surgery), cutting the utero-sacral ligament isn't required. There are enormous studies happening at the moment to evaluate the risk of prolapse but, because it is a relatively new procedure, we don't have hard data. Reports from the surgeons at the hospital I refer into suggest that prolapse is unlikely to be an issue.

What type of hysterectomy?

If possible, you want to have a laparoscopically assisted vaginal hysterectomy or a vaginal hysterectomy, rather than an abdominal hysterectomy. Vaginal hysterectomy is generally seen as the safest way to go. There are no cuts in the belly; the uterus is removed via the vagina.

However, this procedure is not always an option. There are some situations when the uterus is too big, due to adenomyosis or fibroids, or it is technically inadvisable due to previous intra-abdominal scarring or previous surgery or ovarian cancer, in which case an abdominal hysterectomy might have to be performed. This is generally for only a very small proportion of patients these days. Abdominal hysterectomy comes with a higher risk of complications, such as infection, bleeding, blood clots and nerve damage, than vaginal or laparoscopic hysterectomy. Plus, you generally need a longer hospital stay and recovery time and can get more pain and more complications down the track.

Dr David Rosen reports that patients usually say it's the best thing they ever did and often wish they had had it done sooner. So, to sum up, hysterectomy isn't so amazing that it should be given to every woman, but, in the hands of the right gynaecologist, it is nowhere near as awful as many women fear and deserves a proper place in the discussion of options available to you.

What if my low iron is nothing to do with my periods?

Not all low iron is due to heavy periods. If we can't blame your periods, we need to look elsewhere. Iron deficiency either means you're really not eating enough, you're not absorbing iron from the jejunum of the small intestine, or you're losing it somewhere. Committed vegans and vegetarians can struggle to consume enough iron. So it could be your diet. If it's not your diet, your GP is going to sit up and take note, because it's potentially serious. If you have no known gut issues, such as tropical sprue (and you'd know — trust me!), pancreatic cancer or cystic fibrosis, and you're not absorbing iron, it could be coeliac or Crohn's disease. Your doctor will probably run a bunch of tests to look for those conditions. And we always check for the possibility that you're losing iron; it could be from your urine (microscopic blood loss won't be visible to the naked eye), from kidney or bladder problems, or it could be from the bowels. So we will run checks of your poo or even send you to a gastroenterologist to get your guts checked up.

In truth, even when I'm really thorough and check you top to toe, I rarely find a cause of low iron. We don't know why this happens to some people, but you still need to get checked.

How do I fix my low iron?

As well as finding the cause of your low iron — whether excessive bleeding or something else — we have to replace the iron you're losing. There are a few ways we can do that.

Diet

You can simply increase the amount of iron-rich foods in your diet. Red meat (and, to a lesser extent, poultry and fish) contains haem iron. There is also iron in pulses and legumes (think beans, peas and lentils), green leafy veggies (such as spinach, cabbage and broccoli) and tofu, nuts and seeds, but this iron is non-haem. Non-haem iron isn't as easily absorbed by our bodies. If you're a vegetarian, it is very hard to get iron levels up from a low level by diet alone, so I'd see a dietician to get some help. Even carnivores can struggle.

Iron tablets

Iron tablets are cheap and easy to find and use. But because they're non-haem iron, they get absorbed slowly, which means it can take a long while to bring your levels up. Not everyone absorbs iron from their food or from supplements in the same way. Vitamin C increases your absorption of iron, while calcium, fibre, tea, coffee and wine inhibit its absorption. A major side effect of iron tablets is constipation; for many women this can be horrendous and unbearable, and even be a deal-breaker for some. Iron tablets are fine for mild iron deficiency. But many of my patients with perimenopausal bleeding are very, very low in iron and the tablets will just take too long to get them feeling right again. So we need an alternative.

Iron injections

Ow! Looking at a vial of iron, they are *huge*, and most women who have had the injections have found them to be painful. It was actually our old practice nurse, Sister Muriel Baird, a veteran of women's health, who showed me how easy and painless it can be to give iron injections. They have to be given into the gluteus maximus (buttock); she mixes the vial with half a millilitre of local anaesthetic and injects the lot. Few of my patients report pain with this technique. If patients choose this route, we do weekly iron injections of two vials at a time — this is often enough to fix the problem. The downside? The injection technique has to be good. I have patients reporting ongoing pain at the injection site or tattooing (it looks like you have a bruise) over the injection site, which can last a year. This can happen with even the most experienced nurse.

Iron infusion

With this method, the equivalent of 10 vials of iron (or a year's supply by diet) are run into the vein through a drip. Most GPs don't have the infrastructure to do this so I refer to my local infusion clinic, which will take patients with a very low iron level and perform the infusion in a little over 20 minutes. It is not cheap and some people get a mild fever or an allergic reaction from such a massive dose at once. But, once that iron is all in, you don't have to come back each week for more shots and you can chuck your iron tablets in the bin.

You need a good two weeks for injected iron to be fully integrated into your haemoglobin so you are carrying a full load of oxygen again.

Fixing perimenopausal bleeding and giving iron-deficient women iron is one of the most satisfying things I do in my practice. Explaining to these exhausted women that there's a reason they're feeling so tired, and seeing them turn around and feel 10 years younger so quickly is one of the best things I can do as a doctor.

Karen's story

Karen is my age and I've seen her as a patient for years. She's a big-hearted woman with two great kids, a huge circle of friends and a dog she loves. Her periods started getting heavy at age 45. Within two months, Karen had to leave work for the first time when she flooded her clothing. She was mortified. A blood test showed she was incredibly iron deficient, despite eating a lot of red meat, but her pelvic ultrasound at that point was pretty normal. She had no hot flushes at that stage, was a non-smoker, and was in the healthy BMI range. She had a normal pap test, examination and ultrasound. To cover her for both contraception and to lighten her period, I started her on the pill. Within a year that had stopped working. Not only was she having heavy periods again, but breakthrough bleeding as well.

She went to the gynaecologist, who tried a few different things. First she was given tranexamic acid, which basically failed — the periods were still as heavy as ever. Then she had a D&C (for some reason on its own with no treatment added in), which gave her two months' reprieve. By now things had changed and she was starting to get severe period pain as well. It was like the period pain she used to get before having her children, only worse. I ordered another ultrasound; this time it was suggestive of adenomyosis. Maybe it had been there all the time but just not picked up by the initial ultrasound. Regardless, I sent her back to the gynaecologist as she was spending five days out of 26 (the length of her cycle) almost completely out of action. This time the gynaecologist tried her on a progesterone-containing IUD (didn't work) and then she had endometrial ablation (which worked for two months). Now at 50, after five years of this horror, three procedures under general anaesthetic, multiple iron infusions and thousands of dollars out of pocket, she went to another gynaecologist.

She had a hysterectomy. After having feared it, cried about and sought every available alternative, she finally got the definitive treatment. 'I should have done it years ago,' she told me when I saw her last. She's back to running, she just went away for a dirty weekend with her husband and she's really enjoying her work.

A note about too much iron

There is one tiny problem with iron. Other than bleeding, the body doesn't have an easy way to get rid of it if it starts building up. Too much iron isn't great for the body, as the excess iron gets shoved into your liver, heart and pancreas, where it ultimately can (but usually doesn't) lead to cirrhosis, liver cancer, heart-rhythm problems and diabetes.

There is a genetic disease called haemochromatosis, with which people tend to accumulate very high levels of stored iron. But, even for people without haemochromatosis, high iron can still be a problem. One huge study of 32,000 women, whose health was followed for 10 years, was the Nurses' Health Study. It is often quoted because we have accumulated so much data from these 32,000 women. It found that the women with the highest iron levels were nearly three times as likely to get diabetes as those with the lowest iron levels.

And, as I tell my mum all the time (when she tries to force-feed me a steak, citing the argument that not eating red meat isn't natural), heavy red meat consumption is linked to early death, bowel cancer, stroke and diabetes. While on the topic, some people believe it is the excess iron consumption that is the problem. But most people agree the link between heavy red-meat consumption and heart disease and stroke is more likely to be exposure to more saturated fats than more iron.

If it's not my iron, my thyroid or lack of sleep, then why am I *still* tired?

Sometimes we don't find a cause of your fatigue. That doesn't mean you're being told to stop bothering your doctor. As a GP, I can tell you that all it means when you get negative test results is that we don't know why you're exhausted. But we've ruled out some really nasty (and fixable) players. So what do you do then?

So, you wake up feeling exhausted but have a huge day ahead and need your energy and wits about you . . . If you're not exhausted all the time, but just have energy-depleted days, try working through this checklist in case something is helpful.

Drink enough water

Or coffee, tea, low-fat milk or whatever. The Australian National Health and Medical Research Council has stated that as little as 2 per cent dehydration can cause not only fatigue, but also headaches, sluggish mental and physical performance, poor oral health, as well as a higher risk of kidney stones and even some cancers. How much do you need to drink? Well, women need 2.1 litres of fluid a day (any fluid actually; it doesn't have to be water) to replenish what you lose through sweat, breathing and peeing. If it's a hot day and you're sweating more, you'll need to drink more.

For so many women around menopause, drinking plenty means a full bladder and that means wet underpants (see Chapter 4, What the hell happened to my vagina?). So they cut back their fluid intake. Sacrifice your brain for the sake of your bladder? I don't think so!

As you're getting old, you might not recognise the telltale signs of thirst! So keep an eye on your urine (darker means you need to drink more). And, if you feel tired and sluggish, have a glass of water just to make sure dehydration isn't at play.

Perhaps you just don't like the taste of water? (I don't love it, I have to admit.) You can drink any sort of fluid, but juices and soft drinks are packed full of sugar and acids that are bad for your teeth. Water is better. Or tea or coffee without sugar. I like fizzy water so bought myself a little Soda Stream machine and make my soda water each day for work. Or sometimes I chuck in a mint leaf, some ginger or a slice of orange.

No sugary snacks

Not what you wanted to hear? I know that when you're feeling tired, you're often really keen to crack open a chocolate bar and get a quick sugar hit.

Science says that idea sucks. In one of my favourite ever studies, subjects were randomised to either eat a candy bar or go for a ten minute brisk walk when feeling tired. The candy bar group reported feeling increased energy and reduced tiredness immediately after their snack. Plus higher levels of tension! Then, an hour later, they crashed, reporting increased tiredness and reduced energy. The walkers? Well, they had significantly increased energy levels and lower tension than those who were snacking, both immediately and an hour later. The bottom line is that sugar is not a good option for an energy boost, but a brisk walk will be a big win.

Stand up straight!

A nice little American study investigated the link between your posture and your energy levels; 110 university students rated their energy levels, then walked in either a slouched position or with an upright posture swinging opposite arms and legs for two to three minutes. Then they again rated their subjective energy level, swapped movement types and rated themselves again. Slouching made these students report lower energy levels, while the good-posture, arm-swinging walkers reported feeling significantly more energy. The good news was that in changing posture, energy levels rapidly increased.

Ready to hone that posture? Give this a try:

1. Stand against a wall, with the back of your head, shoulder blades and buttocks all touching the wall, and your heels 10cm from the wall.
2. Put a flat hand (not a fist) at the small of your back. If you have good posture, that hand should only *just* fit between the wall and your back.
3. If there's too much space there, pull your belly button backwards towards your spine to flatten the curve in your spine and gently bring your lower back closer to the wall.
4. If there's not enough space at the small of your back to fit your hand, arch your back a little; just enough to fit your hand behind you.
5. Got it? Walk away from the wall while holding that posture. That's a top posture.

As for sitting, it can be very hard to hold a good posture so here are my tips:

1. Keep both feet flat on the floor.
2. Keep your weight evenly distributed between both buttocks.
3. Put your bottom against the back of the chair to keep you sitting up straight.
4. Use a lumbar support if you need to.

If you haven't already, give it a try right now. Whatever position you're in now, try to suck your belly in and pull your shoulders back. Feel any different?

Have a coffee

Coffee, or even just a caffeine-containing tea, can give your brain a decent dose of energy. I resort to this energy hack often! Coffee isn't bad for you; in fact, coffee consumption has been linked to a lower risk of cardiovascular disease (including heart attack, heart failure and stroke), type 2 diabetes, Parkinson's disease, uterine and liver cancer, liver cirrhosis and gout.

The downside is that some people get a bit jittery on it. Some people can get heartburn and some can get mild palpitations, which are annoying rather than dangerous.

Of course, if you don't like coffee, don't force yourself. I just wanted to let you know that, if you like coffee, you can feel pretty pious drinking it, instead of guilty!

What about some long-term strategies to boost my energy?

But quick fixes aren't always what you need. If you're tired day in, day out and your doctor doesn't have any answers . . .

Get enough sleep

Do I sound like a broken record? Despite emphasising how the hormonal events at this time conspire to steal your sleep, I cannot stress enough the link between poor sleep quantity and quality, and fatigue. I know you're thinking: that's obvious. The thing is, when you're tired, your brain goes to water and you don't connect the dots. I don't go a day in my surgery without someone telling me how tired they are. They suspect a medical cause. And when I take a history, the lack of sleep stands out in neon. Make it your priority: I would aim for better sleep before anything else.

Start to exercise

If you already go to the gym regularly, skip this section. But if, like me, exercise is a challenge for you, read on. Lots of my patients are *busy*. Perhaps you are working nine hours or more a day, plus a commute. Plus house work. Plus kids, grandkids and parents. Plus maybe a friend who is going through chemotherapy or a neighbour who just got home from hospital. We are all just so ridiculously busy these days. Add in (for me!) a deep aversion to exercise. I will admit that walking my dogs, Freddy and Ginger, fills me with joy, but let's not call it serious exercise. I doubt my heart rate changes much over the half hour round trip to the park. Other than walking the dogs, the thought of exercise is just horrible. If I get a few rare precious minutes when I'm not working or folding washing, the *last* thing I want to do is run. Or lift weights. So I make every excuse not to do it. The weird thing is, when I force myself to do it, I feel pretty good and always think 'I should do this more often'.

If you're feeling tired and zapped of energy, exercise might feel like the hardest thing to do, because it requires effort when you feel like you have no energy. But it is one of the most effective things you can do to boost your drive. The science is pretty much in. In one review of 70 studies on the connection between exercise and energy, involving almost 7000 people, the link was huge. Over 90 per cent of the studies showed that couch potatoes who started (and finished) a regular exercise program had dramatic improvements in fatigue, compared to those who stayed sedentary.

Fix your allergies

Hay fever and allergy sufferers are often completely exhausted. This is probably due mainly to interrupted sleep, even if you aren't aware of it. Lots of my patients don't connect their hay fever, itchy eyes and wheeze to their tiredness. Try an over-the-counter antihistamine — non-sedating if you need to go to work the next day. The sedating ones can make you feel completely stoned, even the next day if you take it at night. I have lots of patients who have felt 100 per cent better after getting their allergies sorted.

Why am I so bloated?

Bloating is such a crazily common symptom in my practice. And, it turns out, my practice is pretty typical. In studies, anywhere from 15 to 30 per cent of us say we have had some bloating. And that seems to increase around perimenopause; we still don't know why. The good news is that it seems to reduce once you have crossed over into menopause.

When I say bloating, I mean abdominal distension. Many of my patients come in complaining that they 'look six months pregnant'. And yet, studies have shown that the feeling of being bloated doesn't always come packaged up with visible abdominal distension. In fact, the two only occur together in around half the cases of *feeling* bloated!

Bloating sucks. A survey from the US found that over 65 per cent of patients with bloating rated their symptom as moderate to severe. The same study found that 54 per cent of bloated patients said they had had to curtail some daily activity due to their bloating. And, 43 per cent of patients took medication for their bloating.

While we don't fully understand all of the causes of bloating, it is usually associated with irritable bowel syndrome (IBS) — and 90 per cent of people with IBS report bloating.

IBS tends to be a long-term condition that flares up for a period of months from time to time. Stress is one thing that often causes a flare-up. Other theories include a change in the flora (bugs) that live in your large and small bowel. Collectively, the bugs in your gut are known as your microbiome and, while there are 10 to the power of 13 human cells in your body, you have 10 to the power of 14 bacteria in your body! And those cells and those bacteria are in a constant conversation. They influence not only your gut but also your entire body, sending signals out to your immune system, heart and brain.

Diagnosing IBS is interesting. It is what we call a 'diagnosis of exclusion'. There are no tests for it as such but it is what we're left with when we add together your symptoms and the lack of any other diagnosis.

It is an incredibly distressing condition, but, thankfully, has no link to any serious diseases such as cancer or inflammatory bowel disease. It won't shorten your life and it won't cause malnutrition due to poor gut function.

Is the bloating because of my hormones?

IBS-type complaints in women peak in perimenopause, between 40 and 49 years of age. After menopause, IBS rates drop off a lot.

So we're pretty sure hormones play a role. Plus, we have data about HRT and its impact on bloating from IBS. In the UK there is a well-known General Practice Research Database of women aged 50 to 69 years. An analysis of the database found that women who used HRT were more than twice as likely to report having IBS as 'never-users'.

Regardless of your stage in life, management of IBS has improved as more and more evidence emerges about what really works. But unfortunately there is no silver bullet. Here are a few simple ideas that might help.

Keep a diary

This is about your food and drink versus your symptoms. Everyone is different but, after a while, your own individual patterns emerge and you should be able to work out which foods you need to avoid to keep your symptoms under control.

Low FODMAP diet

FODMAPs are types of carbohydrates that aren't absorbed properly in the gut. They've been found to trigger symptoms in people with IBS. Eliminating FODMAPs from your diet can reduce your symptoms by 75 per cent. Given that FODMAP foods include onion, garlic, avocado, gluten and dairy, plus a whole raft of other foods, this diet is pretty challenging. But you only need to go all out for two to six weeks. Then, when all FODMAPs are out of your system and you're feeling better, you reintroduce the eliminated foods one at a time, slowly. This is to isolate which are the culprits for you. Everyone is different and some people can tolerate most FODMAP-containing foods. There are great FODMAP apps to help you.

Mind–body therapies

Managing your stress will help keep flare-ups under control. There's a decent amount of evidence for gut-directed hypnosis, biofeedback, relaxation and meditation for helping manage IBS.

Probiotics

There are a lot of probiotics on the market, all claiming to boost 'gut health'. They are essentially live bacteria that mimic some of the bacteria normally found in a healthy gut. There is some (albeit limited) evidence that some probiotics may improve symptoms of IBS, such as abdominal pain, bloating and gas. The problem is that, because the evidence is weak, we don't know which ones to use, at what dose or for how long. If you find they work for you, that's great. Keep going! Give it eight weeks and then, if you haven't seen a benefit, stop and don't waste your money.

Peppermint oil

Trials of this popular herbal remedy for IBS have produced pretty mixed results. Some studies show that popping it in capsule form can really improve belly pain, bloating and gas. If it's not in a capsule, some forms of peppermint oil can give you horrific heartburn. Peppermint oil seems to be safe. Again, I think it's worth a shot for bloating and bellyache, and if it works keep going. If not, move on!

Can we talk about constipation?

Not all bloating is from IBS. Last week I saw three people with the same problem. All three had severe bloating and abdominal pain. In one case the pain was severe enough to make her go to hospital. In all three cases, tests produced the same results (*major* constipation and nothing else) and last week was pretty typical in my world. All three of my constipated patients were incredulous and suspicious of my diagnosis. But I know as night follows day, that when I see them this week, all three will be feeling lighter, less bloated and in less pain. Let me give you another case study . . .

Tina's story

Tina is 53 and recently went through menopause. She came in with three months of bloating along with a left-sided belly pain that had at first just niggled. Then, over the last ten days, it started to wake her at night and she now described it as severe. It was so severe the previous night that she'd gone to an emergency department, but after waiting for four hours she'd gone home.

I asked her about urine symptoms. None. How were her poos? 'No issues, I go every day,' she told me. No nausea, vomiting; her appetite was good. A bit too good. She had become very stressed at work recently. More and more was being demanded of her with no increase in pay; her boss had some kind of issue where she would be incredibly cold and cutting at times. Then OK for a while, but Tina basically never knew where she stood.

Tina managed her stress through her food. Eating lots of chips, chocolate, ice-cream, crackers . . . The family were getting more and more Uber Eats as her work hours got longer and longer, and she couldn't cook. When I saw her, she'd gained quite a bit of weight and she looked shocking. I got her up onto the examination bed and her belly felt pretty full. Am I being too euphemistic? She felt full of crap.

I quizzed her once again: 'Bowels OK?'

'I go every day,' she insisted, as they always do when I ask! I sent her off for a bunch of tests. Urine, blood, stool, abdominal X-ray and ultrasound.

A week later Tina was back for her results. Like the other patients I saw that week with the same problem, Tina's tests were all plum normal except the X-ray. The result was not the kidney stone Tina suspected but 'significant faecal loading'. That's radiologist speak for massive constipation. Tina was gobsmacked. Like every other woman I see with the same story, she was convinced she couldn't be constipated because of her daily poop.

What should a normal poo look like?

As I told Tina, it's about quality and quantity, not frequency. If you eat a lot, but poo a small amount every day, the maths says you'll be leaving some behind. Which accumulates over time (especially if you miss a day here and there). And down the track you end up like Tina at your doctor's, being tested for what turns out to be a very awkward diagnosis.

So a normal poo should look:

◆ Like a log. Not little pellets, or a bunch of grapes, or even chicken nuggets. Log.

◆ Brown. Not black, red, green or white. Within brown, I'm OK. No need for pics, or detailed descriptions, thanks.

◆ Soft. Poo should come out easily. If it's hard like concrete or runny like diarrhoea, and that continues for more than a week, see your doctor.

Note that frequency is truly variable. Some people go twice a day. Some once every other day. Once you miss two days, your stools will get harder and you'll end up in a constipation cycle.

Fix your sluggish bowels

This is my method for sorting out sluggish bowels, with input from gastroenterologists over the years. First, you need to understand that there is a massive traffic jam in your bowels. To unblock the traffic jam with maximum efficiency, this is my fail-safe checklist:

1. Light diet. Eat like you would after a gastric bug. Low fibre is the way to go; do not send more traffic (fibre) into the traffic jam. Eat white bread, rice, chicken soup, cooked veggies or cooked fruits. No salad or grainy bread, please. Ensure you drink 2.1 litres of fluid a day.

2. Stool softener. We aim to turn a cement brick (poo traffic jam) into a putty consistency to allow the stool to move through the bowels. In kids I use Lactulose, but in adults I like Macrogol. It's a powder that you mix into a drink. Mix it into your tea, coffee or champagne. I don't care! Follow the instructions twice a day until lift-off.

3. Stool lubricant. This is to help the cement brick slide out. I use liquid paraffin. About 40ml after dinner, please. More than one hour before bedtime. Again, do this daily. Until lift-off.

4. Lift off! This is an exciting event or series of events! You'll be utterly amazed at what your body was holding on to and will feel wonderful. Unless you get completely impacted again because you fall off the wagon, lift-off will never happen again. So enjoy it!

5. Post lift-off we need to get cracking with a high-fibre diet. Think grainy bread, baked beans, raw vegetables and whole grains such as oats, quinoa or lentils. Keep up your fluids (2.1 litres a day, please). Keep the momentum moving forward in the bowels.

6. Continue the Macrogol, one dose a day for a month in the fluid of your choice.

7. If you go a day with no bowel movement in the first three months, go back to the beginning and increase your Macrogol, add the liquid paraffin and cut back the fibre until another (albeit much less impressive) lift-off occurs.

The advice above is Gold Plated and deserves awards — it always works a treat.

In Tina's case, I sent her to a gastroenterologist as well. Even though her diet had changed to match her stress levels, she had a change in her bowel habit. And change can mean something nasty in the bowels. The other two women who got their identical test results on the same day are much younger (in their twenties), so I didn't refer them, as bowel cancer in people under the age of 50 is not common. But if their constipation persists despite a good diet and adequate hydration, they'll be off to the specialist, too.

And now that we're on a roll, can we talk about farting?

I'm trying to remember, but I am pretty sure I have never had a patient come in and complain about excess farting. And yet bloating usually comes packaged up with farting. So I'm just going to jump on in and give you some pearls of wisdom! Put down your sandwich and I'll share some fun facts about your bowel gas.

When you're fasting, a healthy gastrointestinal tract (GIT) contains only about 100ml of gas altogether. It seems to be fairly evenly distributed between six compartments of your GIT — stomach, small intestine, ascending colon, transverse colon, descending colon and distal or (pelvic) colon, which includes the rectum. But, let's face it, most of us aren't fasting, so our average gut gas is between 155 and 220ml. Studies have looked at the volume of bowel gas and symptoms of bloating, and they don't match. Bloaters don't have more gas, as far as we can tell.

Where does bowel gas come from?

You swallow a lot of it. Researchers have noted that when some individuals drink, they swallow twice as much air as liquid, especially if drinking through a straw. But swallowing gas is only part of the story. There are five principle gases that together make up over 99 per cent of intestinal gas. Of these, only two — nitrogen and oxygen — are actually present in the atmosphere we breathe in decent amounts. So they're the only two we could have swallowed. The other three intestinal gases — methane, hydrogen and carbon dioxide — come from the bacterial flora in the colon. In other words, your bowel bugs make the remainder of that gas!

How much gas do you pass?

If you're healthy, you'll 'emit flatus' (fart) about 12–25 times per day. And, if you're an average, healthy adult, you'll pass around 2 litres of bowel gas per day. If you don't pass any bowel gas in a 24-hour period, you have a bowel obstruction. Call an ambulance. If someone claims not to fart, then do the same for them. Or call them out as a big fat liar.

For most people, baked beans, soybeans and other legumes will increase the production of hydrogen and carbon dioxide by those trusty colon bacteria.

Smelly versus fragrant

None of the five major fart gases actually smells bad at all. Seriously. The typical aroma of faeces comes courtesy of minute quantities of a few other gases, including hydrogen sulphide, scatols and indoles.

Although less than 1 per cent of gas is stinky, your bowel bacteria produce several sulphur-containing compounds that are extremely stinky. The human nose can detect hydrogen sulphide in concentrations as low as one-half part per billion. That means passing even a very small amount of this gas is unlikely to go unnoticed.

Your farts through the day

Weirdly, we fart most while we are asleep. With the amount of farting done during daylight hours by some people I know, all I can say is: 'God help their partner!'

A few tips to reduce farting

- Eat slowly to swallow less air.
- Increase physical activity.
- Avoid lactose (if you are intolerant).
- Gradually increase fibre in your diet.

Cut back on:

- Talking while eating
- Eating when you are upset or in a hurry
- Using a straw to drink
- Drinking from a bottle
- Sipping hot drinks (let them cool to lukewarm)
- Smoking
- Chewing gum
- Drinking fizzy drinks

- Eating foods containing sorbitol and fructose

- Eating foods you know upset you — perhaps artificial flavouring, caffeine or shellfish

Why have I got so many aches and pains? I feel like an 80-year-old

Aches and pains are often seen as symptoms of menopause. It certainly seems that women get more aches and pains as they age and it often starts around menopause. The aches and pains can be in joints and/or in the muscles.

You need to see your GP to be checked out and not just assume whatever pain you have is due to going through menopause. Back pain, for example, can be a symptom of osteoporosis, probably from fractures in your spine — even if you don't remember having had an accident or falling over.

It's hard to gain statistics about how common aches and pains are during menopause. The massive Study of Woman's Health Across the Nation or SWAN study came out in 2001. This was a study of over 16,000 women around menopause transition across various ethnic groups, places and races in the US. It actually found that 'stiffness and soreness' were the *most* common symptoms of menopause. At 58 per cent, they were seriously common. In the SWAN study this number was higher than those reporting hot flushes, even though the generally accepted number for hot flushes is 75 per cent. To better understand this phenomenon, once again I turned to Dr Terri Foran. She told me she sees aches and pains as being very common among menopausal women, especially in certain ethnicities. 'It's really common amongst Asian women,' she told me. 'Even in the absence of hot flushes, which are far less common amongst Asian women, the aches and pains often drive them crazy.' She pointed me to a number of studies that show body or joint aches and pains are *the* most commonly reported menopausal symptoms in Asian women. And, she pointed out, these aches and pains actually respond really well to HRT.

Despite a fair amount of study showing a link, absolute proof that menopause causes aches and pains doesn't exist. One of the problems is that getting older is linked to a higher prevalence of arthritis and muscle aches and pains, as is being overweight or obese. What can we attribute to menopause and what to the other two phenomena that often occur at the same time? I just think it's interesting that studies in Asian women find that treating the aches and pains with HRT provides relief. So that would indicate that oestrogen plays a role in these symptoms.

I think to assume that you have a painful hip because — and only because — you're around the menopausal stage of life is an error. What if you have arthritis? Or gout? You need to be diagnosed and appropriately treated, so step one is to head to the doctor. But I'm going to assume you have done all of that, and the aches and pains still trouble you. Here are a few things you could try.

Get into a healthy BMI range

We know that being overweight or obese increases your risk of aches and pains considerably. It just makes sense if you're suffering from back, hip or knee pain that you try to put less stress through your joints. See Chapter 7 for tips on weight loss. As a GP I really struggle with telling people who are overweight, and have some arthritis or other musculoskeletal problem, to lose weight. Exercise can be tough when you're feeling stiff and sore. But it will make you feel much less uncomfortable and help you sleep better at night if your back isn't sore.

Exercise

Exercise is hands down the best way to combat chronic (lasting three months or more) aches and pains. It is more effective than acupuncture, physical therapy, massage or non-steroidal anti-inflammatory drugs. This is based on multiple, high-quality trials.

Which exercise? Studies vary from well-known exercises such as walking, cycling, swimming and lifting weights to Pilates, yoga and tai chi. No one is better than any other and the benefits are thought to be as much about changes in the brain around the perception of pain as the actual issue in the back or knee.

Which leads me to . . .

Acceptance

I'm not sure where we've come up with the idea that you should have no pain of any sort. I think it has to do with this idea about what pain is. Doctors used to treat pain as a symptom, or even a warning signal of some underlying problem or disease process. Maybe, in the beginning, pain is a warning sign that something is wrong. But evidence suggests now that once pain lasts longer than a couple of weeks, the relationship between pain and the underlying problem is tenuous at best. But the link is solid in our heads. So pain begets fear that something terrible is at the heart of your pain. And that fear ironically makes your pain worse. That not only leads to an over-reliance on pain medications but also an avoidance of things that hurt, such as exercise. Even if we know from studies that exercise is our best tool to combat chronic aches and pains. You don't need to have no pain; you should aim for manageable pain. And a reasonable amount of pain is something we can come to terms with over time by practising acceptance. Acceptance of pain, acceptance of distress.

Just to put your mind at ease, a recent meta-analysis of painful exercises versus painless exercises for chronic pain found that exercise regimes which included painful exercises yielded statistically significant benefits over pain-free exercises — at least in the short term.

HRT

Dr Terri Foran has extensive experience of positive results of using HRT for chronic pain. There was one study in which the old Women's Health Initiative (WHI) data was analysed. It found that oestrogen-only HRT was linked to a significant reduction in reports of aches and pains. Now, I have spent a goodly amount of time ripping the headlines of the WHI study apart — but it does have some fantastic data. Having said that, not a lot of doctors would prescribe HRT if aches and pains were the only symptoms you had. But chat to your doctor, especially if you are from an Asian background, because the evidence in your ethnic group is much more compelling!

Is there anything I can do to help my bone health?

From about age 30, your bones and their muscles start to lose their integrity and strength. The loss of bone density just speeds up intensely in women after menopause. As a result, bones become more fragile and are more likely to break due to osteoporosis. What can you do to protect them?

Exercise

When it comes to your bones, use them or lose them. Weight-bearing exercise and resistance exercise that put some stress through your bones are essential to build healthy bones and repair brittle bones.

Don't smoke, and only drink at healthy levels

Excess alcohol (in the case of osteoporosis, it's any more than two standard drinks a day) and smoking have both been linked to an increased risk of osteoporotic fractures. While we're depriving you of things you love, you might need to cut back your caffeine a bit, too; the maximum seems to be 250mg of caffeine a day. To put that into context, there is 80mg of caffeine in an espresso coffee — so three coffees is your limit — and about 30mg in a brewed tea. I totally bust that amount every day of my life, so you'll get no judgement from me!

Get adequate calcium

Having a diet low in calcium (and here I am thinking about a dairy-free diet) increases your risk of osteoporosis. We ideally like you to have at least 1000mg of calcium per day, which is about three serves of dairy a day. You can also get calcium from non-dairy foods, such as dark green veggies (e.g., kale and broccoli). Ideally eat them raw or just cooked for a couple of seconds. Oily fish such as sardines and salmon work well, too. Five tins of sardines a day ought to do it! Some milk alternatives have calcium added — you just need to check the labels as they're all so different. If you simply can't handle dairy, you might need a calcium supplement. Take two or three 500mg tablets max and take them with food.

Get enough vitamin D

This interesting little vitamin comes in very few foods, is fortified into some foods, or taken as a supplement. The main source is actually sunlight. You make vitamin D when ultraviolet rays (UVB) from sunlight hit the skin and trigger vitamin D synthesis in the skin itself. You've probably heard about it, but let me explain why it's so important. Vitamin D helps your gut absorb calcium, regulates the amount of calcium and phosphate in your blood, and helps build quality bones. Without enough of it, you risk osteoporosis. We also know that UVB exposure and associated production of vitamin D reduces the risks of 15 forms of cancer, and we have some confidence (but not certainty) that it, in fact, reduces the risk of all cancers.

We used to get most of our vitamin D from sun exposure. But with all the fear of skin cancer (and rightly so) we're seeing more and more deficiency. In fact, a 2005 study estimated that every year in the US between 50,000 and 63,000 people die prematurely from insufficient UV exposure. This results in an economic burden of US$40–56 billion per year. That, compared with an estimated economic cost of US$6–7 billion a year associated with excessive UV exposure from things such as skin cancers. Not a pretty measurement unit, but a stark rebuke to the message that we should totally protect ourselves from UVB. And one of the problems is that we just haven't worked out the optimal exposure. The closest we've come to the establishment of a recommended UVB dose is 'in moderation' or to 'avoid tanning or burning'. There has been a wave of enthusiasm for vitamin D supplements, but the data to confirm that they help with disease prevention (as compared to normalising your vitamin D levels through a bit of sun exposure) is pretty weak. But I take vitamin D supplements because there's no real evidence they don't work and my work hours are too long to be able to rely on getting enough sunshine.

Stay in a healthy weight range

Being underweight increases your risk of osteoporosis. Probably because you're not putting enough stress through your muscles and bones. Being obese (with a lot of fat cells, as opposed to having a high BMI due to stacks of muscle) is also linked to increased risk of osteoporosis.

Get diagnosed sooner rather than later

A DEXA scan of your hip and spine will usually pick up reduced bone density. In the US, screening with a DEXA scan starts at age 65. In Australia, screening starts at 70 (for men and women). We would start scanning you earlier if you had a high-risk condition such as coeliac disease, rheumatoid arthritis or premature menopause. Chat to your doctor about the best time to start having scans.

Get treatment

If you find out that you already have osteoporosis, there are many medications you can use. Chat to your doctor about the best option for you. HRT is awesome for bone health, but there are other specific medications for osteoporosis as well.

Why are my breasts aching?

No chat about aches and pains is complete without discussing aching breasts! I'm going to focus more on perimenopause here because this becomes a very common symptom during the years of hormone hell. How common? Well, I only saw 15 patients yesterday and two of them complained of aching breasts. Hey, sisters, I can relate. I've gone from an A cup bra to a Double D, and my breasts ache so much I would sometimes like a straitjacket to hold them in place.

So, we are not alone. In fact, back in 1987, a study published in the *British Journal of Surgery* found that 69 per cent of women attending a breast cancer screening clinic said they experienced breast pain. Yet breast pain is poorly studied and the advice given to women by doctors is frankly woeful!

Here's what we know about mastalgia (the medical word for sore breasts). According to academics, mastalgia generally falls into three types. Cyclical breast pain, as the name suggests, happens in a typical cyclical pattern, usually around the period. It's the most common form of breast pain and tends to hit women aged between 30 and 50 years. Both breasts are equally painful but the ache tends to be worse in the upper outer parts of the breasts. Hormones (especially oestrogen) are blamed. This is because of the cyclical nature of the pain, rather than because we have the foggiest clue about *how* your hormones cause the pain. We know progesterone (the hormone that surges in the second half of your cycle) causes enough fluid retention to push you up an entire bra cup size.

The second, and in my experience in my surgery the most common, form is non-cyclical breast pain. You guessed it! It has no relationship to the cycle and often only affects one breast at a time. I see this often. The examination of the breasts is rarely revealing, and often, just as we start doing scans, the pain just goes away. Unfortunately, it tends to come back again, either in the same or the other breast.

I will admit we know close to nothing about this type of breast pain, except that it tends to hit women between the ages of 40 and 50. Benign breast problems like cysts and fibroadenomas (benign tumours) can be the cause. Breast cancer is unlikely to be at play here. Out of interest, only one in 200 women who see their doctor about breast pain have breast cancer as the cause. But still, even a remote chance is enough to make me urge you to get a GP check-up. If you have nipple discharge or a lump, make it an urgent check-up. Just a small note here: sore breasts can be a sign of pregnancy! If you're not in established menopause, you might want to buy a home pregnancy test and rule that out.

The third type is non-breast breast pain. You feel pain in the breasts but it's actually coming from another body part. The heart, for example. OK, that is rare. But given we know how common it is for heart disease to be unrecognised in women until it's too late, this is one not to be missed. Chest-wall pain from excessive coughing, a massive gym work-out or lifting something heavy (called Tietze's disease) is another cause, as is oesophageal pain, from reflux for example. So a trip to your doctor is one of my top tips for managing breast pain.

The doctor will ask you a bunch of questions, mainly to pinpoint or lower suspicion of any sinister cause of your breast pain, such as breast cancer. Dimpling of the overlying skin and bleeding from the nipple are worrying. Lumps are a less reliable sign of breast cancer, as they are most often benign and just cause everyone, including your doctor, grief until the negative results come back.

You'll be given a thorough examination and then we often do an ultrasound, with or without a mammogram. Mammograms are less reliable in women under the age of 50 because the breast tissue itself is very dense, making reading the mammogram trickier for the radiologist.

Let's jump ahead here and assume you're all clear on the cancer front, and what you have is a diagnosis of mastalgia. So now what we want to know is how to stop your breasts being sore. These are my recommendations.

Keep a diary

Especially if your breast pain is cyclical, understanding your patterns of pain will be helpful in planning ahead and managing the problem.

Make sure you have a decent bra

If you have anything more than a C cup, a sexy little number is not going to be comfortable at that time of the month or whenever your boobs are aching. The good news is that simply getting a better-fitting bra will fix breast pain in 85 per cent of women. You might want to get some help; I think professional bra fitters are amazing but it's getting harder to find them, especially if you live in a rural area or want to shop online. If you're fitting a bra on your own, look for wide shoulder straps and a firm grip. Sports bras are designed to minimise jiggling, so initially you can feel like you're wearing a corset. But push on.

If getting a whole new set of lingerie is going to break the bank (bras are ridiculously expensive), then grab a couple of cheap crop tops and wear one (or even two) over the top of your existing bra.

Just to bust a couple of myths: underwired bras don't give you cancer. Wires don't compress the breast and lock in toxins or cancer-causing chemicals. That's been pretty well studied now, so wear any bra you find comfortable. It's all down to personal preference. And you can wear a bra to bed. Again, it won't give you cancer or lumps or build up toxins. Many of my patients wake up from the pain when they accidentally roll over onto an engorged painful breast in bed. They get incredible relief from wearing a bra to bed.

Bust your stress

While we know for sure that breast pain is not a neurotic condition or just psychosomatic, we also know from studies that stress makes it worse. Busting stress helps reduce breast pain, which is a win–win.

Wait it out

Most studies find that breast pain goes away once you hit menopause. Unless you go on HRT, in which case it can continue.

Anti-inflammatory medications

Grab an over-the-counter non-steroidal anti-inflammatory gel or cream. Think of Diclofenac. Not only do studies support its use, but in my experience it's a massive winner. There are no significant side effects reported in medical journals but popping cold gel on your boobs three or four times a day in winter can be less than appealing. So we have other options . . .

You can take your anti-inflammatory medication as a tablet. Studies find it's equally effective as the gels, but has more side effects such as tummy upsets, especially if you don't take it with food, plus high blood pressure, kidney damage and even a higher risk of stroke. Don't fall off your chair — the last two are really only a problem if you take high doses every single day. Just take them when you have pain and you'll likely feel a lot of relief without a high risk of side effects.

Diuretics

The rationale of using a 'pee pill' is that breast pain caused by fluid retention due to a progesterone surge in the second half of the cycle should, in theory, be nixed by losing some of that excess water. But it hasn't been studied and there are side effects such as low blood pressure due to water loss (through all that peeing!), so there's a growing consensus that they are not a good option for breast pain.

Try other meds

Danazol, Tamoxifen, Goserelin injections, Bromocriptine and Toremifene are all effective but there are reported side effects that most women and their doctors find unacceptable. From growing a beard and developing a deep voice to period cramps, weight gain and cystic acne, hot flushes and aches and pains, dizziness to severe constipation, the side-effect profile of this group of drugs is too nasty when we have such simple over-the-counter medicines available.

Evening primrose oil
A much beloved home remedy, this has actually been extensively studied and found to be 'an expensive placebo treatment'. In studies it did no better than a placebo, albeit with side effects limited to stress on your wallet!

Vitamins B6 and E
Long touted as cures for breast pain, sadly the evidence doesn't stack up for these guys. I'm a fan of getting your vitamins from your dinner rather than an artificial capsule, but, other than an unnecessary expense, at least there aren't many side effects.

And, finally, some good news!
For years, doctors used to say you had to avoid coffee to stop your breasts aching. Thank goodness we can kick this myth to the kerb. It has been well studied now, and we can say with confidence that cutting out coffee will not do anything to help your poor boobs. Ditto, steering clear of caffeine in tea and colas (although I'm not advocating any soft drinks here!).

Can HRT cause breast pain?

This is super common. In fact, one worrying study found that, even on low-dose HRT, 53 per cent of women got mastalgia, compared with only 6 per cent of placebo users. We don't know why this is.

If this happens to you, please chat to your doctor. I usually switch women from traditional HRT, containing oestrogen and progestogen, to Tibolone or a TSEC, a combination of oestrogen and Bazedoxifene that nearly always fixes the problem. If the dose of HRT you need to keep the flushes at bay is higher than the dose of Tibolone or the TSEC, we can add an anti-inflammatory as well.

Why am I so itchy?

Menopause and itchiness are commonly linked. When you think about all of the effects of menopause and sudden loss of oestrogen on your skin, it's not really surprising. In the absence of oestrogen, your skin not only loses much of its structural support, such as collagen and elastin (see Chapter 9, Make me look like Helen Mirren), but it also loses a lot of its moisture. This is from a combination of losing sebum, the skin's natural oil, and hyaluronic acid, the natural, moist, gel-like fibre that supports the structures within the skin.

The result? Itching and even formication — a sense of insects crawling around under your skin . . . No, that's not a joke. I had heard of this happening when heroin users go cold turkey, but it turns out menopause and even perimenopause are triggers, too. If you get formication, as well as treating the underlying skin issues, see a doctor for some specific medication to deal with the problem.

Let's just deal with the itch first . . . Around menopause, the pH level of our skin changes and becomes less acidic. With this change, skin becomes more sensitive. So you're more prone to rashes and easily irritated, itchy skin.

Dermatologist Dr Eleni Yiasemides often sees itchy skin among menopause-aged women. Her best advice is to use a bath oil in the shower and a really good moisturiser. She's not prescriptive about which one. Having skin that is less dry will usually make the problem better for most women. Avoid soap because of its tendency to dry out the skin.

Over-the-counter antihistamines can work wonders, too, she adds. Creams containing urea can be great for recalcitrant itch. If that doesn't help, head to a dermatologist for a thorough once-over, a proper diagnosis and maybe some prescription medication.

The itch can specifically affect your hands and feet. *Keratoderma climactericum* gives you a skin build-up on your palms and soles, especially your heels. It starts at menopause and can make your feet super itchy, but it can even make walking painful. It is admittedly more common in obese and hypertensive menopausal women. Dr Yiasemides advises women with this condition to use a combination of salicylic acid and urea as a heel balm. She advises women to avoid pedicures. 'All the scrubbing makes your skin form more keratin so it actually makes the problem worse,' she says.

TIRED, BLOATED AND ITCHY
THE BOTTOM LINE

Tiredness becomes a huge issue for many women around menopause time. For many this is caused by lack of sleep. Between 40 and 60 per cent of women get insomnia during perimenopause and menopause. Lifestyle changes and some medications and complementary treatments can help.

Tiredness can be caused by other issues, such as iron deficiency caused by heavy periods. If you are losing more than 80ml at each period, there is help you can seek from your GP or specialist to make your bleeding lighter.

Many women complain of bloating and irritable bowel syndrome during perimenopause. This also usually disappears once full menopause is reached. Often it's caused by constipation, even if you think you are 'regular'.

Aches and pains in our bodies are a common complaint of women around menopause. We can try to combat them through lifestyle measures such as exercise. HRT seems effective in stopping them.

Many women have sore and aching breasts around menopause — the link has not been established but there are lifestyle changes you can make to manage this. It tends to stop after menopause, unless you are taking HRT.

Reduction in oestrogen causes changes in your skin that can lead to itchiness and sensitivity. There are easy over-the-counter treatments for this.

CHAPTER 7

WHERE DID MY WAISTLINE GO?

When I was 47, my dad died. It was pretty traumatic, I can tell you. Anyway, within a year, along with picking up some hot flushes, I had gained over 10kg, drifting outside my healthy weight range for my height for the first time in my life. I felt sluggish, looked rubbish and my cholesterol and blood pressure went up. I know how it happened and it wasn't my hormones. Wine o'clock had become established in my house. My husband, who is a junk-food addict, was bringing home lots of 'treats' to have after dinner and I was doing close to no exercise. I work long hours and have a pretty solid commute (over an hour to my surgery). My mum, who is generally slow with reprimands, said: 'You'll want to lose some weight before you hit menopause. After that it's really hard.'

Mum's not wrong. Between the ages of 45 and 55, women gain on average 700g a year. And, certainly among my patients and friends, it's really tough to budge it.

When I was studying medicine, we were taught that in order not to gain weight, energy in had to equal energy out. And people who gained weight were greedy and lacking self-discipline, or were grabbing a sneaky pack of chocolate biscuits at 2am. Thankfully, it has now been proven that your weight is not simply a mathematical equation of calories in versus out.

Instead, it is associated with the whole problem of altered physiology. So let's look at the culprits that change your physiology.

The case against disappearing oestrogen

Oestrogen definitely helps you burn fat. There is plenty of scientific evidence that losing oestrogen gives you extra fat accumulation, and that accumulation is disproportionately in the abdominal area. This central fat build-up comes packaged with insulin resistance (disrupted sugar metabolism with weight gain as a side effect) and cholesterol problems.

From science experiments, we know that oestradiol can stop a chemical called lipoprotein lipase in your fat cells. This is an enzyme that basically converts fatty acids from the bloodstream into fat cells. And in rats oestrogen curbs your hunger.

In one 1997 study, 875 women were randomly assigned to get three different HRT combinations or placebo. After three years, the women on any HRT had gained an average of around 1kg less than the women on placebo. They also had on average 1.2cm less increase in their waist circumference and 0.3cm less increase in hip circumference. Women gained more in their hips if they drank alcohol and gained more in their waist if they did less exercise at the start of the study.

We know that in studies oestrogen increases physical activity-related energy expenditure. In other words, if you have oestrogen on board, you burn more energy during exercise. But you do have to exercise! However, the studies are a bit inconsistent, with some finding oestrogen plays no role at all.

The case against hunger hormones

Discovered only in 1999, ghrelin, the hunger hormone made in your stomach, turbocharges your hunger and decreases the amount of energy you burn up. In a healthy body, after a meal your full stomach stops making ghrelin and you lose the desire to eat. This is disrupted in people with obesity, who just stay hungry and overeat. Go on a diet or lose weight, and your blood levels of ghrelin after a meal increase. What we don't know is whether the problems with regulating the hunger hormone cause obesity or the other way round.

Leptin, derived from the Greek word *leptos*, meaning 'thin', has the opposite effect. It is made by your fat cells, reduces your hunger and makes you use up more energy. Bottle this one for me, please! Now, before we all go searching Google for Ukrainian websites selling leptin supplements, let me warn you that the science behind leptin is like Swiss cheese. For example, obese people have higher blood levels of leptin than skinny people. Scientists are still baffled by this and wonder whether obese people become leptin resistant? Or whether leptin resistance *causes* obesity? Regardless, put your wallet away until we understand it better.

There is one more hormone that plays a role, more in metabolism than hunger per se. Adinopectin is another peptide that increases fat metabolism and stops the liver producing sugar. Scientists are looking at turning it into a therapy for obesity but are just not there yet.

The case against getting older

The science is there. Women, without doubt, gain weight at 'midlife', but multiple studies consistently show that weight gain is due to age, not menopause. Two things happen at once. First, we lose muscle mass as an inevitable part of the aging process. Muscles are metabolically very active so that loss means we burn fewer calories, both at rest and when we exercise. On top of that we tend to sit more and move less. These two factors conspire against us and explain why we may gain weight with the same diet and exercise routine that previously kept us looking trim.

The case against sleep deprivation

Along with hot flushes and night sweats comes massive sleep disturbance. Being tired can destroy your ability to adhere to a healthy diet and regular exercise routine. Who craves celery and steamed fish when you're running on hardly any sleep? You want a quick energy hit — chocolate and crackers! Going out for a brisk walk or meeting a girlfriend for a Zumba class is especially unappealing if all you want to do is flop on the couch and watch TV after a long day. The result? Research has found that adults who get four or less hours sleep a night have an increase in their hunger and appetite. And, to make matters worse, what you crave when you're running on empty is processed, calorie-dense carbohydrates. No surprise then that sleep restriction and obesity are linked in studies.

The case against insulin

The hormone insulin is the 'drug' that Type 1 diabetics need to inject into themselves to stay alive. When you eat some sugar your pancreas (up in the top part of your abdomen) releases insulin. Insulin is the key that unlocks the doors in the cells to allow sugar to enter and fuel the cell with energy. If there's no insulin, the sugar cannot enter the cell. Insulin makes your body scavenge for excess sugar and turn it into fat for a rainy day, while also switching off fat burning so your body uses sugar instead. Having lots of insulin around is fantastic in a famine, or in a week-long winter blizzard in a cave.

In some of us, probably through a combination of genes and lots of food without enough exercise, the insulin locks get rusty and don't work as well. The insulin is there aplenty but it's less efficient in opening the doors to allow sugar into the cells. This is insulin resistance. Insulin resistance has been linked to the development of diabetes, cardiovascular disease and Alzheimer's disease. Multiple studies have linked obesity with high insulin levels and insulin resistance. The jury is still out about the chicken and egg situation at play here. Does obesity and a bad diet make you insulin resistant or does insulin resistance make you gain weight? There is some evidence that insulin is a weight-gain accelerator. Metformin, a medication used to treat diabetes and polycystic ovaries, partly by improving insulin sensitivity, has been shown in studies to help with weight loss. I'm pretty convinced!

The case against being a couch potato

Here is a statistic you might find fascinating: resting energy expenditure accounts for 60–75 per cent of total daily energy expenditure. And resting energy expenditure declines by approximately 420kcal/day in postmeno-pausal women compared with premenopausal women.

I have no idea why this happens around menopause. It has been linked to the loss of metabolically 'active' muscle mass. But, while scientists try to confirm that this slowdown in resting metabolism does, in fact, happen at menopause and then work out why, we'd be remiss if we didn't look at your activity levels, too. Scientific studies confirm that women do seem to stop moving as much at perimenopause when they're exhausted from insomnia. Then, when they're having hot flushes and are hot, the idea of exercising is pretty unattractive. If you run and wet your pants, you'll think twice about running. If you've been up all night flushing and sweating, you'll be too exhausted to move much.

The case against anxiety and depression

We've known for a while now that experiencing stress, anxiety or depression is strongly linked to being heavier and having a worse diet. But the question is: does comfort eating make depressed people fatter? Or does being over-weight impact on your mood? Do certain unhealthy foods make you bigger *and* more depressed? And, most importantly, can changing your diet help your mood *and* your weight?

Scientists have been trying to tease this out a bit. Comfort food gets its name for a reason. Eating certain foods leads to dopamine production in the brain. This dopamine activates reward and pleasure centres in the brain. Some of us will subconsciously chase this dopamine high by just eating a particular food that triggers dopamine release over and over again until we eventually can't read the brain's signals of satiety and hunger. Take chocolate . . . Science tells us that chocolate has a strong effect on mood, generally increasing pleasant feelings and getting rid of tension. If I'm hot and sad, I can see chocolate's many attractions.

But it's about more than just making dodgy food choices when you're feeling low. Studies show that people suffering chronic stress tend to have more central abdominal fat that is driven by excessive systemic cortisol levels.

Why has my shape changed?

Hormonal changes in menopause do result in a change in body composition, with increased fat and decreased muscle. They can cause fat to settle in your abdomen rather than your hips, thighs and buttocks. Hello belly! That is both your belly subcutaneous fat (the fat that sits under the skin around the belly) and visceral fat (fat around the organs so your waist expands without wobbling under the skin). This happens even if you don't change your physical activity or total body weight.

Now, as well as looking somewhat less attractive, this change in shape also puts you at risk of some chronic diseases — diabetes, for one, as well as higher cholesterol and heart disease. In turn, diabetes also increases the amount of fat that sits around abdominal organs, such as the liver. This fat, called perivisceral fat, causes your waistline to expand disproportionally to the rest of your body (like your thighs and hips) and will also independently increase your risk of related diseases such as heart disease.

But I'm fat and happy

I'm saying: you're lucky; it's rare. For so many women, there is an emotional burden from stacking on pounds during midlife. It can take its toll on your self-image, your relationship with your partner and even your sexual function. But if you've gained weight and feel great, I still think you ought to try to budge a bit of weight.

Believe me when I say I don't care what you look like. I don't judge your clothing choices and am in no position to throw stones from my glass house at your wobbly thighs. But this is about health. Obesity is a major contributor to diabetes, cardiovascular disease, dementia, some cancers (endometrial, breast and colon), depression, sexual dysfunction, urinary incontinence and musculoskeletal disorders, especially osteoarthritis.

How can I budge the menopause weight?

When it comes to losing weight, there is no silver bullet. The science hasn't changed. The most effective way to lose weight and keep it off is to eat a healthy, low-calorie diet and be more physically active. We all know it isn't always that easy. So, I am going to share with you my greatest tips of all time for controlling your weight. Weight is a daily battleground for me, so I'm not judgemental of anyone. But here is what works for me.

Write it down

You are eating more than you think and moving less than you think. For sure. There was an iconic study published in the *New England Journal of Medicine* back in 1992, which is still incredibly relevant today. This was a study of people who were obese, eating 1200 calories a day and not losing weight. In other words, 'diet-resistant' people. They (along with a control group of people who were managing to lose weight) had close monitoring of their diet, their exercise and a whole stack of tests to assess their metabolism. The hypothesis was that these people had a 'slow metabolism'. So here's what the researchers found: the metabolism in the two groups was identical. But the 'diet-resistant' people were under-reporting their eating by 47 per cent and over-reporting their exercise by 51 per cent. Not to be sneaky, but just because getting it wrong is common and easy. But difficult to combat.

From the available evidence, it does seem that writing down every bit of food you eat does help with weight loss. Certainly, in my experience it is one of the cheapest and most effective tools I have to help someone with their weight. The problem is actually doing it. I find that snacking makes people stop journalling and, with it, stop losing weight.

Eat less

I don't want to be too glib about this but you do need to consume fewer calories to lose weight. Studies show that most women should consume 1200 to 1500 calories a day to lose weight. Do that and you can expect to lose, on average, 0.5 to 0.75kg a week. I'm not a big fan of calorie counting and, to be honest, I find you can get yourself into a tizzy of obsessive-compulsive behaviour if you go too far down that track. Rather, you just need to calculate the big picture of what 1200–1500 calories looks like. For example, if the average steak is about 200g, you can expect to take on

270 calories from the steak. Add in a single baked potato (93 calories) and a dressed salad (21 calories) and your daily calories are starting to run out, on a diet dinner. A bag of chips is over 500 calories, a hot cross bun over 300 calories. I'm only saying this to point out that sticking to a low-calorie diet means not eating an awful lot. If you're feeling hungry, don't give in to the need for food. You won't die by having one less spoonful of pasta for dinner.

Are you really hungry?

Often when you eat, it's not because you're hungry. You eat out of habit; you eat because you're bored or stressed. Eating is not only a necessity for survival but also a great source of pleasure. As long as you are eating mindfully. To explain all of this, I turned to a colleague I very much admire.

Ginette Lenham is my go-to nutritional counsellor. She addresses that nexus between grief, trauma, relationship and family conflicts, body image issues, depression and anxiety with your eating. I met her years ago when doing research for a book about polycystic ovaries. From the moment I met her, I loved everything she had to say about dysfunctional eating. I had sent countless women to dieticians, who would helpfully advise them not to have a packet of chips, but instead have some celery sticks and hummus. Sorry? If there is anyone out there battling their weight who doesn't realise they shouldn't eat chips, I haven't met them. People with weight issues don't need to be patronised or fat-shamed. They need to be supported with practical ideas they can actually implement. Ginette gets all of this and has helped many people wrangle their control back. Here are Ginette's tips for using mindfulness in battling weight gain around menopause.

First, take notice of whether you are eating because you are actually physically hungry or for reasons that have nothing to do with hunger, such as:

- You may be eating because the clock says it's time to eat.

- You may be eating just because everyone else is eating.

- You may be eating because it looks yummy and you just want to have it.

- You may be eating out of ritual, such as popcorn or choc tops at the movies.

- You may be eating because you are at a social event and you feel uneasy — eating gives you something to do.

- You may be eating because you are bored and it helps pass the time.

- You may find yourself cooking for a family even though offspring have moved out and therefore you eat more than you need.

If it is just occasionally that you find yourself eating in these situations, it will not be a problem. But paying attention to the cues and motivations for eating should help you become much more mindful of your eating patterns and allow you to acknowledge if there are any habits that could be changed.

And second, take notice of your satiety cues. Many of us eat way past our 'full' point. You don't need to eat until you are full. Eat until you are satisfied. Get in touch with your body and be more mindful of every mouthful so you don't eat past your mark. Enjoy each mouthful. Pay attention to your food and how it feels and tastes. It will make you eat more slowly and it will help you eat less.

Drink a glass of water before a meal

If I get dehydrated, I need something to feel better — that something often ends up being food, despite the fact that what I *really* need is water. If I remember to drink water instead of eating, I often feel better *and* don't eat as much. It could be the effect of being better hydrated. Studies have linked drinking less than a litre of water a day to slower metabolism, less fat burning and reduced weight loss. Hopefully we'd all drink more than 1 litre of fluid a day, so it often comes down to when.

One 12-week randomised placebo-controlled trial compared drinking two glasses of water before a meal with visualisation exercises — basically imagining a full stomach. The study was done on obese adults. Both groups lost weight but the water drinkers lost significantly more weight. This is a simple, easy and achievable weight-loss strategy that any of us can use.

Do a detox

If you are going to reduce the size of your waistline, we need to take a tour of your pantry and all the secret locations where junk food lives. These need to be thoroughly detoxed but not the way you think . . . My 'detox' is not the same as most naturopaths'. I simply mean getting rid of the food stuff in your life that is making you fatter, more sluggish and more miserable.

I am cringing as I share my dirty little secret: I'm a jelly snake addict. If I buy them I'm a goner. A whole pack goes in less than 10 minutes. Nobody is a flawless eater, and if you need to lose weight and you have problems with self-control (like a human being, rather than a kale-bot), junk food *cannot* be in your house. If it's there and you know it's there, you need the self-control of an Olympic athlete to resist it. It's hard enough to resist the endless birthday cakes at work and the dessert when you go out for dinner. Having rubbish at home is a disaster. Throw it away. Seriously. And you don't need to have junk food on hand 'just in case someone comes over'. If I come over to your place and you start serving cakes and chocolates, now *I* have an issue. Can you bring out some carrots and cheese instead? Just make a pact with other family members that it doesn't enter the house.

A side note about the other type of 'detoxing'

The premise behind dietary 'detoxing' is rubbish. Those who peddle detoxes will tell you that your body is swimming in a toxic sludge fuelled by chemicals, the environment and your food and that these toxins overwhelm your body, causing everything from fatigue (hands up if you don't have that?) and headaches, to belly fat, cellulite, wrinkles and cancer. I get frustrated by the pseudoscience that surrounds these claims, so let me explain what *really* happens between toxins and your body.

Humans come ready-packaged with a brilliant detox kit — the liver. Together with your skin and kidneys, it does all the detoxing you will ever need. Lots of my patients have been told by a naturopath that they have 'a sluggish liver'. This is a sort of catch-all diagnosis. I'm not saying that sluggish livers don't exist. In fact, cirrhosis of the liver (which is usually eventually fatal) makes the liver very sluggish indeed. If you have cirrhosis I am pretty sure that you will know it. You won't just feel a bit tired: you will be bright yellow from jaundice, waterlogged from retained fluid and hardly able to move through exhaustion. You can also become psychotic, as toxins build up in your brain. Does this sound like you? No, I didn't think so . . . Your liver is fine and it's handling your toxins just fine.

I'm not completely anti-detox. Because, like many crazy pseudoscientific ideas, buried below all the drivel was once some very good advice: drink enough water. So many of us are walking around very under-hydrated. You will feel better just by being well hydrated, so I'm happy with that advice. Similarly, eating more of the good stuff such as fruits and vegetables is a no-brainer. Ditto, cutting out processed, high-sugar foods. But the expensive supplements are worse and useless ('colon hydrotherapy' in particularly is a potentially dangerous activity).

The Rule of France

If you're lucky enough to have strolled along the banks of the Seine, or anywhere else in France for that matter, you will probably have been grateful for all the tourists. Because the locals can make you feel like an elephant. On my visit, I was fascinated by the fact that the average patisserie (and it feels like there's one on every corner) has sold out of pastries by lunchtime and yet the French all look like catwalk models. And don't look for joggers: they're pretty thin on the ground! I thought maybe it was just genes, but after a while I worked out something: eating is a French celebration; the French all sit down for their meals.

So I invented the Rule of France for myself. If I don't sit down at a table and put my food on a plate, I can't have it! No more grabbing from the biscuit barrel at work while I boil the kettle; no more eating crackers standing up while I cook dinner. No more standing at the sink eating leftovers. I have to set the table, put the food on a plate and eat it slowly and mindfully. You will also find this helps guard against the under-reporting of your eating (page 209).

The Rule of the US

My patients always have a chuckle when I tell them to eat like an American. So let me explain: I'm not telling you to add salt and sugar to everything and supersize your meals. Instead, I like the American concept of starting the meal with a salad. I might not *love* the type of salad they eat, but the concept of filling up on salad and veggies is great. We know we should all be having five serves of vegetables a day (a serve is half a cup of cooked veggies or 1 cup of raw). It is hardly surprising that only 4 per cent of us manage that.

When I ask patients what they had for dinner last night, the answer is often 'chicken' or 'roast lamb'. The veggies, such as they are, are very much a sideline. But we know that it's the meat or fish that should be the added extras to the vegetables. One easy way to do that is to make an entrée of salad like the Americans (or even just chop a plate of raw veggies). Start with that for your evening meal. And, once everyone has had a plateful, move on to the rest of the meal. It works!

Check your fluids

When you are battling your weight, sadly you need to cut out any drink that is not water, tea, coffee or the occasional alcoholic drink. I know that can be very difficult but I want you to think about the number of calories you consume when you have a drink such as fruit juice. There are about 6 teaspoons of sugar in the average glass of orange juice. And 9 teaspoons of sugar in a can of soft drink. That sugar contributes to unnecessary calories you just don't need. There is nothing in fruit juice that you need — substitute one glass of juice for a couple of whole pieces of fruit, and in doing so grab yourself the same vitamins, with added fibre and antioxidants from the skin that is removed during the juicing process.

As for soft drinks, they just pack on calories with zero nutritional benefit whatsoever. Lots of my patients drop large amounts of weight just by cutting out soft drinks.

Thinking about diet soft drinks is also evolving. Most doctors have traditionally considered them a better option than the full-sugar varieties, but this is all changing. Studies have found that consumers of full-sugar soft drinks have the *same* risk of diabetes as those drinking diet soft drinks. And we know that regular consumers of diet soft drinks tend to be fatter and have more abdominal obesity. This certainly raises the possibility that the sugar isn't the only issue with soft drinks. Here are some other potential problems:

- Too much artificial sweetener can affect your gut, giving you flatulence, diarrhoea and tummy pains. That might make you crave simple carbohydrates such as crackers and rice.

- Artificial sweetener might disrupt the gut microbiome. Researchers are looking at how this could also contribute to weight gain.

- Long-term high consumption of diet soft drinks is linked to lower levels of activity in the part of the brain that gives you a feeling of satisfaction from your food. So you might compensate by eating and drinking more.

- Diet soft drinks seem to prime the brain to crave sweet foods, thus sabotaging your diet.

Wave goodbye to wine o'clock

When Dad died, I started drinking. It might not have been a lot by other people's standards but, instead of drinking a glass of wine once or twice a week, now we were opening a bottle every night. One glass of red wine has 125 calories, two glasses has 250 calories. A gin and tonic is around 145 calories. Given that to lose weight we generally recommend a total of 1200–1500 calories a day, the calories from just two glasses of wine can add up to more than a fifth of your daily budget.

A major study of the relationship of alcohol reduction in the context of weight loss revealed some interesting results. Cutting back on alcohol did lead to more weight loss, but not from the alcohol calories per se. It was more about preventing episodes of overeating and binge eating, especially in people with poor impulse control. So the researchers concluded that cutting back on drinking was a great idea, but not because wine is 'fattening'.

Get organised

Losing weight is not about being told by a doctor that a tuna salad makes a better lunch than a bag of chips and a Coke. But it is a lot about being organised. You need to have the good food in the house or you will have no choice but to order in takeaway for dinner. If you haven't brought a healthy snack to work and you get hungry, then you'll probably scoff down an entire piece of birthday cake if it's on offer. So I recommend buying a stack of veggies that will keep for the week: capsicums, snow peas, cucumbers, cherry tomatoes, or whatever you like. Have them washed and ready to take with you to work as a pre-prepared meal or snack. For me, a little reusable lunch box of vegetables (with a pickled cucumber) is a great lunch, with a hard-boiled egg or a small tub of cottage cheese and a couple of wholegrain crackers. If that sounds boring, you're right! But it does the job. It takes me no time to prepare and guarantees I'm getting enough veggies each day. I also keep small boxes of nuts in my drawer at work in case I'm still at the surgery at 7pm. Try having your vegetables delivered if you can't get to the shops. And frozen vegetables are just as nutritious as the fresh stuff and work well for a quick, easy dinner, so always have them in your freezer.

Keep it all in perspective

I love food. I love cooking, but I love eating more. I know there are people who really couldn't care less what they eat. They skip a meal because they were busy doing something and forgot to eat. Forget a meal? How do you do that? They don't watch cooking shows, read cookbooks, swap recipes or really enjoy any meal all that much; not in the way they enjoy a good run, movie or a great book. Those people often have no issues with their weight because they just don't get enough satisfaction from food to be bothered binging on it.

But there are other people who aren't eating much for different reasons. It's not that they're disregarding food; it's the culture of deprivation and restriction. See if you can pick these people . . . they love food but they can't eat any of it because they're on some special diet. It's protein shakes, or palaeo, or carb-free, or clean eating, the Candida Cleanse or one of the other regimens that some genetically blessed Hollywood personality has attributed their good looks to.

Whether you're detoxing off coffee, alcohol, sugar, fat, artificial colourings, flavourings, carbs or taste, the sacrifice is *too high* once it starts stealing the fun from your life. When you can't go out for dinner with your partner, you can't celebrate your mum's birthday, or have a glass of wine with a girlfriend, the cost of your eating regime is *way too high*. Food, rightly, has a place front and centre of our society and culture, and no diet should come between you and seeing the people you care about. (Plus, so many of the strange and extreme diets I hear about these days sound more like self-punishment than a serious attempt to make a long-term healthy change to your life.)

My philosophy is the 80:20 rule. What matters is what you do most of the time, rather than all of the time. When you do have a chocolate, some cake or some chips, my rule is: enjoy it! There should never be guilt. If you think you'll feel guilty after eating something, then don't do it. In my case, let's go back to my guilty confession about those jelly snakes. If I buy and then open a bag, I'm done for; so, I either don't buy them, or I buy them with someone, take out a couple and then give the bag to my workmates. I'm not controlled enough to just have two and save the rest for another day. But those two I have before I give away the bag are just fantastic!

Exercise

I am already feeling guilty as I write this. Can I just blurt out a confession before we start? I hardly exercise. I do enjoy it but I don't get the time. I have a rule that if I work less than 12 hours a day, I exercise, but that's rare. Well, the odd Sunday. I'm working on it! Like you, I'm on a journey to better health and my workload is a thorn in my side. Guilt about my completely sedentary life is a daily event.

There are plenty of reasons to exercise: it has myriad benefits for mental and physical health. But we've known for a while that exercise alone won't make you lose weight. The theory behind the exercise–weight loss disconnect used to be that you get hungrier after exercise and often eat more than the calories expended during your work-out. Studies have shown that's simply not true. Not only does exercise *not* drive increased energy consumption, but it doesn't even drive up hunger!

So what's going on? It seems that for those of us who struggle with our weight, we feel so virtuous after a gym session or a good walk that we're entitled to a reward! So we make the wrong food choices. Plus, studies show that we often overestimate the number of calories we've burned during a work-out and underestimate the amount we can eat to neutralise the exercise effect. The bottom line is that if you're exercising for weight loss, it will only work if it comes with a low-energy-dense diet and judicious control of the amount and type of food you eat.

Guidelines globally recommend 150–175 minutes of exercise a week. Any exercise will do as long as it gets your heart rate up a bit. For example, brisk walking or some other aerobic activity, such as dancing. Resistance exercise such as squats, boxing, weights and push-ups increase the amount of lean body mass you have. That is going to increase your basal metabolic rate and energy expenditure.

What about medications to give my belly a nudge?

Let's get this out of the way — medications aren't an *alternative* to lifestyle measures. They're an addition, and are only helpful *if* you have the lifestyle stuff sorted out, too. Having said that, if you are obese (BMI over 30) or have a BMI over 27 plus a weight-related medical problem, such as diabetes or high blood pressure, you certainly qualify for a helping hand from a medication. I have had some amazing success for my patients using many of the medications below. Generally, medications will help you lose 5–10 per cent of your body weight.

Metformin

Metformin is a drug traditionally used for type 2 diabetics to lower their sugar. It has three mechanisms of action: it decreases the production of glucose in the liver; it decreases the absorption of glucose from the intestines; and it improves the sensitivity of cells to insulin. Some research points to a potential fourth role, which is improving the profile of the bugs in the gut microbiome. This better bacterial profile seems to improve metabolism.

Metformin is a bit of a wonder drug. It plays a role in controlling sugar levels in diabetics, but also prevents diabetes in people whose sugar levels are abnormal but not high enough to be labelled diabetes.

Metformin helps with weight loss for diabetics and for women and girls with polycystic ovarian syndrome. But for people with obesity but neither of these conditions, it is a less certain bet. The interesting research area for Metformin is in people with high insulin levels, due to insulin resistance, but with normal sugar levels. It has been successfully trialled in adolescents but not yet in adults; regardless, many endocrinologists use Metformin for adults with insulin resistance diagnosed by a blood test. Right now we just don't have the evidence to use it in overweight and obese people across the board.

Liraglutide

This injectable (yes, injectable — as in you give yourself a needle in the belly every day) medication started life as a diabetes treatment with a side effect of weight loss. Now repurposed for weight loss in anyone, it helps to reduce hunger and also slows down your gut so you feel full more quickly and for longer. It is highly effective as a weight-loss medication but has some pretty intense side effects. It causes nausea, vomiting, gastro-oesophageal reflux and constipation (I have had patients abandon this drug as they simply cannot tolerate it), and it is insanely expensive.

Phentermine

This drug is as old as the hills. It slows down the entire gut so you feel full for longer, and also reduces hunger cravings. Side effects can also be intense: dry mouth, constipation, nausea, anxiety and insomnia are the main ones. It can't be taken by anyone with uncontrolled high blood pressure. I have prescribed this quite a bit over the years and it works, but it can only be used for three months at a time and the side effects can be off-putting.

It can also be combined with Topiramate (a traditional epilepsy medicine with appetite loss as a side effect), which improves its efficacy for weight loss. As well as the Phentermine side effects, we can add change in taste. It also causes birth defects, so can't be used if you're pregnant. (Mind you, if you're planning a pregnancy, I guess you're unlikely to be reading this book.)

Naltrexone plus Bupropion

This drug combines two medications: Naltrexone, which is used to treat alcohol and drug dependence; and Bupropion, which is used to treat depression or help you quit smoking. Together they make you feel less hungry or full sooner. And they probably help battle food cravings, too. This has a long list of possible side effects: dry mouth, constipation, headache, insomnia and nausea. Liver damage and high blood pressure are two of the slightly more dangerous ones. Having said that, in my experience it often works to get off a quick 10kg.

Orlistat

I'm listing this only in the interests of being thorough — it is not one of my favourite medications. It basically stops your gut from absorbing fats, which stay in the bowels. (It does not act on sugar and carbs.) Side effects are tummy aches, nausea and farting, plus it causes liquid 'anal seepage', which is exactly the way it sounds. You would need to take a multivitamin pill with this, because a lot of vitamins come from fat in your diet.

HRT

Women who receive HRT tend to be leaner and have less central obesity. But HRT still isn't given for weight loss alone; that would be a side benefit of taking it for control of menopause symptoms. HRT seems to protect you against type 2 diabetes; although Metformin would be a better choice if it were for this specific purpose only.

What about weight-loss supplements and home remedies?

I have to brace myself when I delve into the absolute disgrace that is the world of weight-loss supplements. The claims are unconscionable, the prices outrageous, and close to none of these products do anything for your weight. Statistics on this are staggering. More than 30 per cent of people who have made a serious attempt at weight loss have tried supplements.

If there was a silver bullet for getting rid of excess bottom and belly fat that didn't require diet and exercise, I'm pretty sure we wouldn't have an obesity problem. No supplement can be mixed with a glass of Fanta and bucket of fried chicken, and lead to your fat melting away. Below are 'the good, the OK and the ugly', with appropriate Gwyneth ratings.

L-carnitine

This is the one weight-loss supplement I would potentially describe as 'good'. This derivative of an amino acid transports long-chain fatty acids into the mitochondria, the engines of our cells, so they can be burned to produce energy. It then turns around and extracts the waste products that build up after the energy-burning process and removes them from the cell. Our bodies make some, and we get the rest from food — mainly animal products such as meat, dairy and eggs. A large meta-analysis of L-carnitine supplements found that, when combined with diet and exercise, L-carnitine supplements saw a loss on average of 1.3kg more than in people taking a placebo. The benefit seems to wane over time, though. Personally, I am not sure that 1.3kg extra weight loss is worth the cost of the supplement. I found them online for around $40 for a month's supply. Woah! But if you like the sound of it, go for it. And, if you're thinking about this seriously, check out Chapter 8 for some added brain benefits that might tip the scales. One Gwyneth for the cost.

Chromium supplements

The metal chromium, apart from looking great on your bumper bar, seems to be involved in carbohydrate, fat and protein metabolism. Back in the 1960s, chromium-deficient animals were shown to have insulin resistance; supplements helped reverse this, but true chromium deficiency is pretty rare. Scientists have shown (from hair samples) that chromium levels go down as we age. Could this be why we gain weight as we get older? Unfortunately, a comprehensive review of 24 studies of chromium on body mass and fat distribution found no real benefits. Chromium does seem to be pretty well tolerated, but it can interact with your medications so chat to your pharmacist about it. Two Gwyneths.

Apple cider vinegar

One of my patients weighs around 150kg. She told me about a year ago she had decided to follow the advice of an Instagram influencer to drink a tablespoon of apple cider vinegar before each meal to help her lose weight. She asked me what I thought of the idea, and this is what I told her.

The science to back up her strategy is a little shaky. Studies in mice do show that vinegar can improve their metabolism and reduce the amount of fat they store in their bodies. There was one human study I could find: 150 obese Japanese people drank a kind of cocktail containing 0 or 2 table-spoons of apple cider vinegar each day. After three months, the vinegar drinkers had lost 700g while the people whose cocktails contained no vinegar gained 200g. Four weeks after the trial had ended, everyone was back to square one.

There was one other small study that found drinking a little vinegar before eating made you feel fuller after eating. The same study also found this fullness was because the vinegar caused nausea!

Downsides? It can make you feel sick in the guts and its acidity can harm your teeth if you don't take care to rinse it off with a chaser of water. But otherwise, if you like it, don't let me dissuade you. One Gwyneth.

By the way, my patient lasted two weeks and then couldn't handle the vinegar. She's still on the diet roller-coaster.

Green tea

To be honest, there is practically no evidence that green tea, packed with caffeine and antioxidants, helps you lose weight. There are a couple of deeply flawed studies in mice. But human trials of green tea, either as a drink or as a supplement, have yielded some pretty pathetic results. Having said that, if you like the taste of green tea and it hydrates you, there's no real issue with it. Zero Gwyneths.

Coconut oil

This is huge on Instagram. Coconut oil has ended up on a virtual pedestal as a one-step healer for everything from a wobbly bottom to heart disease. Studies don't support it for weight loss — by that I mean it *does* work in studies for weight loss *when combined* with a calorie-controlled diet and exercise, but not more than diet and exercise alone. Not enough studies have been done to assess the effect of consumption of coconut oil on the heart and the rest of the body, so experts suggest keeping its use to a small amount. And 'small' is yet to be defined. One Gwyneth.

Green coffee beans

This is one of the most popular supplements for weight loss in the world. The proposed magic ingredient is cholorgenic acid, which is removed from the coffee bean during the roasting process. Together with the caffeine in the coffee bean, there is some evidence that this ingredient does help improve carbohydrate metabolism. And in one smallish study of overweight women (all younger than 45, mind you), 12 weeks of instant coffee with green coffee beans led to around 3kg more weight loss, and loss of more body fat, than standard instant coffee. However, that was combined with diet and exercise again.

There are not many side effects here. So, if you like instant coffee and you like the one with green coffee beans, it's fine to switch. But there is no strong science on it. One Gwyneth.

The master cleanse

This is a strict diet where all you consume is water with added lemon juice, water, cayenne pepper and maple syrup! You read that correctly. You drink this combination for a period of three to 10 days — that makes it a fad diet to me. It sounds bad for your teeth, and bad for your energy levels — you will be hangry for a short time and then regain the kilos. It's a big no from me: two Gwyneths.

Garcinia cambogia

No googling of weight-loss products would be complete without mention of this shamelessly ineffective supplement, a tropical fruit also known as the Malabar tamarind. It is claimed to reduce appetite and block the body's ability to make fat. Endorsed by Dr Oz, it is totally proven *not* to work at all, not even a little bit. It is seriously expensive and comes with enough gastrointestinal side effects to make you wonder if you've picked up a nasty virus. This gets three Gwyneths from me, just for being cruel. How can anyone sell this stuff and sleep at night?

Yohimbe

A Yohimbe is a tall evergreen forest tree, native to south-western Nigeria, Cameroon, Gabon and the Congo. The bark contains the medicinal compound yohimbine, which is widely promoted for weight loss. It's also popular with men with erectile dysfunction. Studies of yohimbe for weight loss have found no evidence to support its use. But wait till you hear the side effects: high blood pressure, anxiety, agitation, rapid heartbeat, heart failure, heart attacks and death. So you'll see why I am a little down on this one. Plus the overharvesting of this tree is making it an endangered species. Three Gwyneths.

Ephedra

Also known as ma-huang, this is one of those herbal stimulants that used to be fairly ubiquitous in herbal weight-loss products. It's now banned by the American FDA because of its side effects, which include mood changes, high blood pressure, irregular heart rate, stroke, seizures and heart attacks. No thank you. Three Gwyneths.

Isn't there anything new being researched for weight loss?

Probiotics

Probiotics are 'good' bacteria that should, in theory, help with a whole range of health and weight issues driven by problems with your gut bugs. The recent theory that gut microbiome influences metabolism started when researcher Peter Turnbaugh showed that if you transplant intestinal bugs from obese mice into skinny mice, the skinny mice become fat.

Studies in humans show that obese people have fewer of one bug (bacteroidetes) and a generally lower bacterial diversity (range of gut bugs) than lean people. It's this low diversity of bacteria that is also linked in studies to more body fat, higher cholesterol, a tendency towards diabetes and a general state of inflammation in the body. Our high-sugar Western diet increases the amount of a bacteria called firmicutes, which is strongly linked to obesity and reduces those beneficial bacteroidetes. A low-calorie diet that results in weight loss seems to increases the relative abundance of bacteroidetes. Changes in bacteria in the gut happen as quickly as in 24 hours. There are a few theories about how gut bacteria affect weight:

- The gut bacteria of obese people may simply be more efficient at extracting energy from food than those in the intestines of lean individuals.

- Bacteroidetes produce short-chain fatty acids (SCFAs) from foods. A greater diversity of gut bugs is linked to more SCFA production. These SCFAs, such as acetate, butyrate and propionate, seem to help repair the intestinal wall, keeping you feeling full and reducing your hunger.

- The SCFAs butyrate and propionate have been shown to reduce food intake and are linked to a lower risk of obesity and insulin resistance in mice.

- Inflammation in the body generally has been linked to obesity. We know that less diversity of bacteria is linked to more inflammation.

So, could probiotics be the answer to obesity? In 2016 a large meta-analysis took place (when researchers look at all the individual studies that have been done and compare and collate the findings). There had been five trials in humans and all of the probiotics were some kind of lactobacillus combo, rather than bacteroidetes, the bug we most want to promote in the guts if battling obesity is the game plan. The studies used these probiotics in varying doses, amounts and delivery systems. The good news is that they're safe and didn't have any major or serious side effects. The bad news is that the probiotics we have at the moment didn't work for weight loss. However, it is such early days. The microbiome theory is so recent that we haven't had time to do enough clinical research yet. I suspect it is going to come, so watch this space.

Pickles, fermented foods, kombucha and other prebiotics

So if we can't change your gut bugs for the better, perhaps we can use fermented foods and drinks such as kombucha (a very trendy fermented tea) to grow your own 'skinny gut bugs'? Microscopic bugs added to these foods use enzymes to alter some of the food components. Lots of cultures use some sort of fermenting process of food groups from dairy to vegetables, fruits, meat and fish. We're talking about pickled cucumbers and kimchi and even yoghurt — and they've been around as long as human civilisation. Societies have fermented foods to make them last longer, taste better and for health benefits.

Early evidence suggests that the fermentation process can make certain vitamins more 'bioavailable' when they are partly broken down by the microbes — B vitamins, including folate, riboflavin and B12, as well as vitamin K2 seem to fit the bill here. And fermented foods seem to deliver beneficial bugs directly to the human gastrointestinal tract. Evidence is growing that these fermented foods can help you prevent metabolic problems, such as diabetes.

In terms of weight, studies are a bit thin on the ground. One study found that eating yoghurt protects you against obesity. But, then again, this was true of eating dairy across the board. So how much of this was the yoghurt and how much the dairy? I'm going to say that in terms of having evidence to support fermented foods for weight loss, at this point we aren't there yet. But I feel they're going to be included in nutrition charts in the future as more evidence emerges. If you can eat a couple of yoghurts and pickles a couple of times a week, I'd call that a win for your body.

And what about weight-loss surgery?

If your BMI is 40 or over, losing just 5–10 per cent of your body weight mightn't be enough. The evidence for bariatric surgery in this group is actually excellent. The problem is that it is expensive, you need a specially trained surgeon to do it, and no surgery is without complications. I don't plan to go into the ins and outs of surgery here because it's something you'd need to discuss in depth with your GP and specialist. Let's just say that unless it comes packaged with diet, exercise and fixing your emotional eating, it will not be a silver bullet.

And once I've lost the weight, how can I stop it coming back?

Research shows that, sadly, around half of all patients who manage to lose significant amounts of weight are back to their baseline weight within three to five years. This is heartbreaking . . . you starve yourself, give up sleep-ins to attend the gym, and forgo parties and champagne just to end up back at square one.

So how do you avoid this? We know that those of us with good social support, who get constant counselling, and those who do 200–300 minutes of exercise a week are more likely to keep the weight off. So it seems logical to keep exercising even when you don't feel like it. See a counsellor, if you can afford it, and connect with friends and families who bring positive energy to your life. After all, it's the emotional eaters among us who are more likely to regain that lost weight. I introduced you earlier to nutritional counsellor Ginette Lenham. Here are her top tips for emotional eaters:

- You might realise you are self-soothing with food, but it's important to know what the causes are of your need to self-soothe. Address these difficult emotions, rather than using food as a bandaid without knowing why you feel emotional.

- Some of the emotional triggers in menopause that can lead to emotional eating might be dealing with the loss of fertility, changes in significant relationships, body image, weight gain, employment challenges, caring for aging parents, loss of sleep and more.

- Once you can label the emotion, see if you can find another meaningful activity that would calm you instead of eating. Maybe a walk, music, having coffee with a friend, having a bubble bath, booking a massage, watching TV or reading a book. Perhaps seek professional help to talk through your struggles.

- If food has been your best friend for a long time, addressing emotional eating can be more challenging. Can you identify the emotion — is it loneliness? Fear? Anxiety? Boredom? Or personal conflicts? The best way to change from emotional eating in response to the situation is to acknowledge the feeling, name the feeling, feel it, and ride out the urge to eat in response to it. This will feel challenging in the beginning. However, over time you will feel more in control.

WHERE DID MY WAISTLINE GO?
THE BOTTOM LINE

Most women do gain weight around menopause time, and oestrogen loss plays a role.

The weight is more likely to go on around your middle.

Being overweight is often upsetting and usually bad for your health.

There are lots of great strategies for losing weight but they all involve changes to diet and exercise. Sadly, there are no silver bullets.

Emotional eaters tend to regain weight if they lose it — so if that's you, there are lots of reasons to be kind to yourself and get help.

CHAPTER 8

THE SHARPEST TOOL IN THE SHED

This chapter is personal for me. Daniel's father, Louis, died of dementia. By the time I met him, the dementia had well and truly set in. He was a happy man, but never really understood what was going on around him. When he died, he was immobile, blank and couldn't speak or feed himself. This was devastating for Daniel, who just adored his dad. He described him as witty, with a towering intellect, fiercely ethical, charming, slightly quirky, fluent in several languages, widely knowledgeable and loving. That is exactly how I would describe Daniel.

Daniel and his brothers talk a lot about preventing dementia happening to them. We have studied all sorts of remedies and great hopes, and I am happy to share them here. Oh, and as well as being brilliant, charming, witty and ethical, Daniel is vague, forgetful and disorganised — just like he was in his twenties. He calls it charming; I'm not sure, but it's certainly nothing sinister.

Dementia is a topic that starts to weigh on the minds of menopausal women, too. Many of us are now caring for parents or in-laws affected by dementia — a stark reminder of our own brains' vulnerabilities. So many of my patients come in, worrying that their brains are turning to water — they're forgetting things, they're losing things and they're worried the dreaded process has started. Statistics reveal they are not alone. At least during peri-menopause, the vast majority of women report memory problems.

Approximately 15 to 20 per cent of people aged 65 or older have mild cognitive impairment (MCI). People with MCI, especially if that MCI impacts on their memory, are more likely to develop dementia than people without it. But it's not inevitable. It looks like 10–15 per cent of people with MCI get dementia each year. Researchers are still grappling with what triggers that transition so that we can prevent it happening.

Does my brainpower really decline around menopause?

Yes, it does. Sorry. There are only a few studies of brain performance around menopause that start on women *before* they enter menopause proper. But two out of three published longitudinal studies say the decline in brain function *starting* around the time of menopause is real.

Certainly during perimenopause, women often say they're getting forgetful. If you test these women, they do indeed show a decline in processing speed and memory for verbal material. Studies confirm there is a high correlation between complaining that your brain is feeling soggy and doing worse on objective cognitive testing.

So is this changing hormones or old age? What's to blame? Probably both.

Oestrogen and brain health

There are both oestrogen and testosterone receptors throughout the brain. But being precise about the role of hormones in brain health has a few problems. Studies have found that oestrogen enhances the ability of nerves to grow into new parts of the brain and form new connections. It also helps with the formation of memories. Oestrogen protects against injury and death of nerve cells in experiments designed to replicate exposure to nerve-killing toxins such as poisons and strokes. It also seems to protect against the accumulation of a protein called beta-amyloid that builds up in Alzheimer's disease.

Oestrogen enhances several neurotransmitter systems, including acetylcholine, serotonin, noradrenaline and glutamate. Acetylcholine is important in memory.

Oestrogen also enhances both your verbal memory and your 'executive function'. The term 'executive function' started as a business metaphor: your executive function is like the CEO who monitors all the departments so that the company works efficiently and smoothly. So executive function wraps up planning and organisation, and then the execution of those plans.

Functional brain-imaging studies have revealed that oestrogen helps brain performance when women are doing cognitive tasks.

So, if oestrogen has all these amazing effects on the brain, it stands to reason that less oestrogen would lead to reduced brainpower. But why does this happen?

It could just be hot flushes. Apart from driving you crazy, hot flushes also seem to contribute to memory difficulties in midlife women. Studies have shown that hot flushes cause significant physical changes in your brain in the hippocampus. But, as you now know, hot flushes aren't necessarily related to *low* oestrogen levels. What I find fascinating about the relationship between hot flushes and cognitive function is this: in a sample of women suffering from moderate to severe flushing, the flushes correlated significantly with poor performance on memory tests. But, only the flushes that could be detected with a range of skin sensors and the like. And they didn't necessarily closely match the way the women *felt*. In fact, the frequency of *reported* hot flushes by the study participants was not related to memory performance at all! This was backed up with changes in neuro-imaging studies — it's the actual flushes that impact the brain function, rather than the feelings of flushing.

Testosterone and brain health

Testosterone is also likely to play a role. How do we know? We have located testosterone receptors in the brain, and there are some small but interesting studies to refer to. For example, in premenopausal women, higher levels of testosterone in the bloodstream predict better mathematical and spatial skills. And, in elderly women, higher blood testosterone levels seem to be linked to better verbal fluency and performance at memory tasks. In postmenopausal women, higher levels of DHEAs, the testosterone precursor made by your adrenal glands, have been linked to better executive function, memory and concentration. Randomised controlled trials of testosterone supplements suggest boosted brain performance. In menopausal women, you don't get the nosedive in androgen levels that you do with oestrogen; it is a slower, steadier decline that is more related to age than menopause per se.

So is it a combination of hormones and just getting older?

Alzheimer's disease accounts for 60–80 per cent of all cases of dementia. And, statistically, women are twice as likely to get Alzheimer's as men. The theory is that both age-related changes in brain function and hormone changes (the gradual drop in testosterone and sudden drop in oestrogen at menopause) contribute.

The brain is so complex — all those different tiny little parts that influence the way we feel, remember, think, calculate, move and speak. As you get older, certain parts of the brain shrink, especially those important for learning and other complex mental activities. In certain brain regions, communication between neurons (our nerve cells) becomes less efficient. Blood flow to and inside the brain slows down. And finally, inflammation, which occurs when the body responds to an injury or disease, increases inside the brain. All parts of the brain, especially those structures supporting memory, are highly sensitive to any kind of stress, partly due to their high demand for oxygen.

So, the changes in the brain that happen with aging can affect mental function, even in healthy people without a diagnosis of dementia. Remembering things, learning new skills and problem-solving can all become harder.

As I am writing this today, we have no remedy for dementia, and it is not clear when or if an effective treatment will ever be developed, despite many pharmaceutical companies working to find one. So the focus has been very much on interventions in people who already have 'pre-dementia' conditions such as mild cognitive impairment. There's early evidence that some interventions might stall the progression of cognitive decline. Currently, we think MCI might be the final point at which intervention can be effective.

What lifestyle and diet changes can I make to prevent cognitive decline?

Exercise

This is a bit of a recurring theme, huh? Hands down the best evidence exists for exercise. Fitter people have bigger, better-functioning brains and they get less dementia. A meta-analysis of randomised controlled trials looking at the relationship between exercise and brain function, especially cognition, did show improvements in attention, processing speed, executive function and memory among older adults doing various exercise regimens. Most experts agree that physical activity is an excellent preventative measure against cognitive decline.

Specifics around whether aerobic exercise versus strength training, yoga or tai chi has the most beneficial effects on cognition, and how much you need to do, are still being nutted out in various studies. But I would suggest half an hour a day of an exercise you enjoy. From ballroom dancing to surfing, or just going for a walk. Whatever you are most likely to do and stick to. For me, my personal trainers are Freddy and Ginger, my beloved dogs. Taking them for walks ticks many physical and emotional boxes for me.

Control the hot flushes

Completely separate to the idea of taking HRT for brain health is to do something about your hot flushes. Controlling them might just be the key to helping your brainpower. In a tiny pilot study, a technique called stellate ganglion blockade was used to control hot flushes. The better the improvement in the flushes, the better the improvement in memory performance. It's an early trial, so more work needs to be done.

Socialise

I'm not sure everyone realises the power of socialising with neighbours, friends and family members for brain health. Studies show that an increase in 'social engagement with the surrounding environment' is linked with growing new blood vessels (angiogenesis), increasing the connections between neurons (synaptogenesis) and the creation of new neurons (neurogenesis). We still don't really know how, but socialising seems to improve your self-esteem and reduce your stress. Lots of the formal studies of socialising took place on people with already established dementia. This condition is so isolating, and loneliness is so pervasive among dementia patients, that it is not easy to extrapolate the findings across people with MCI or those who are looking to prevent cognitive decline altogether. But, most experts agree, socialising is a good idea at every stage for optimum brain health.

Change your diet

Ole! Add some Mediterranean flare to your diet. You've probably heard of the Mediterranean diet, based on the cooking styles of Greece, Italy and Spain. It is a whole way of eating differently more or less permanently, as opposed to the sort of short-term diets you find in magazines or online. It is based mostly on plant-based foods, such as fruits and vegetables, whole grains, legumes and nuts. Other key elements include olive oil, and other healthy fats such as avocado, probably a glass of red wine a night and lots of fish (especially oily fish). Red meat appears only a couple of times a month! Off the table is too much unhealthy fat. The Mediterranean diet is also linked to lower bad cholesterol (LDL), less heart disease, less Parkinson's disease and possibly less cancer, including breast cancer.

Based on both observational studies and randomised trials, the Mediterranean diet seems to have some serious brain-boosting power. Research suggests a Mediterranean diet not only slows age-related cognitive decline in older men and women, but also reduces the risk of MCI progressing through to full-blown dementia or Alzheimer's disease. Plus, it seems to prevent MCI developing altogether.

If only we could isolate the one or two elements of the Mediterranean diet that do the heavy lifting in protecting brain function . . . We have no idea which they are — so you have to adopt the entire thing!

With a bit less evidence behind it, it seems that the DASH (Dietary Approaches to Stop Hypertension) diet also works to prevent dementia. Specifically formulated to treat high blood pressure, this is based on reducing processed food and salt, and increasing whole foods, aimed at increasing your magnesium, potassium and calcium. Think fruits, veggies and dairy. The DASH diet also throws in fish, poultry and legumes, plus a handful or so of nuts and seeds a few times a week. Meat, saturated fats and sugar are kept to a minimum.

More or less dairy?

A Japanese study of 303 older Japanese people who were followed for 17 years found that consumers of the highest amount of milk and dairy had less Alzheimer's disease than non-dairy consumers. This followed a highly reported study by the University of Kansas Medical Center that got equally positive results. It was funded by the National Institutes of Health as well as the US Dairy Research Institute and found that dairy consumers had higher levels of glutathione in the brain. Glutathione is an antioxidant that helps prevent damage to brain cells. There is emerging evidence that low glutathione levels might be linked to dementia.

But these things are never clear-cut. From observational studies, it seems that eating lots of high-fat dairy might *increase* the risk of dementia. It could be the saturated fat, but we don't know for sure.

The bottom line is, if you like low-fat dairy, it is a good choice for your bones. And might, possibly, help your brain. If you're a dairy avoider, there's no need to take it up for the sake of your brain. Regardless, high-fat dairy such as high-fat cheese and ice cream should be a treat food.

A glass of wine

So this is some good news: light to moderate consumption of alcohol has been linked to a lower risk of dementia. The benefits for dementia might be a side effect of the benefits to the cardiovascular system, and therefore the arteries supplying the brain. But moderate intakes of alcohol seem to also reduce inflammation, increase the good cholesterol (HDL) and increase blood flow to the brain. It might even have some antioxidant effects. At this stage, what we can say is that if you like a glass of wine with dinner, feel free to continue. If you don't, there's not enough evidence to say you should take it up.

A glass of wine is not half a bottle. Excessive alcohol consumption and binge drinking (which is only four standard drinks on a single day — and a standard drink is usually far less than we pour ourselves!) increase the risk of developing dementia. The National Health and Medical Research Council's *Australian Guidelines to Reduce Health Risks from Drinking Alcohol* recommend limiting alcohol intake to no more than two standard drinks on any day.

And, if breast cancer is your fear, remember research shows that drinking just three alcoholic drinks a week gives you a 15 per cent higher risk of breast cancer than teetotallers. And the risk of breast cancer goes up by a further 10 per cent for each additional daily drink.

Fermented foods

We met these cool and trendy foods when we discussed bloating and gut bacteria. The idea behind fermented foods is to encourage the growth of beneficial bacteria in the gut. But they might have added benefits. Early research indicates that the fermentation process improves the activity and bioavailability of the food itself. One recent study found that short-chain fatty acids, which are the chemical by-products of the intestinal bacteria enhanced by fermentation, actually help streamline your metabolism and seem to enhance the function of your brain. We are not yet sure how, but it's early days for the research. I love pickled veggies and yoghurts so I'm happy to believe they're good for everything — but if you hate these foods, don't worry too much. At this stage there's no hard evidence they're necessary for brain health or any other health whatsoever.

Blueberries

Well, is this ever a 'superfood'? Oh, by the way, 'superfood' is a marketing term, not a scientific one. There is a little bit of evidence to support the idea of eating blueberries as brain food. We already know people who eat enough fruit and vegetables get less dementia. But in animal studies, blueberry supplementation enhances memory and motor performance. The magic ingredients in blueberries are anthocyanins, which are also in mulberries, bilberries and blackcurrants. Studies show that these anthocyanins enter the brain after you eat blueberries, but we don't know what they do there. A study by the University of Cincinnati of a grand total of nine older adults with MCI found that drinking wild blueberry juice for 12 weeks improved memory. If you like blueberries (and can afford them!) then keep going. By the way, the same anthocyanin punch is packed whether your blueberries are fresh or the slightly cheaper frozen variety. If they're not to your taste or not in your budget, don't worry.

Get enough sleep

I don't need to tell you how being sleep deprived makes you foggy in the head. There's increasing evidence that chronic sleep deprivation can contribute to cognitive impairment. A good night's sleep, with plenty of deep sleep, helps your brain clear beta-amyloid, the protein that has been linked to Alzheimer's disease. So experts have theorised that if your body doesn't get enough good-quality sleep, beta-amyloid might build up in the brain. Evidence for the theory is now emerging. In one small study, losing just one night of sleep led to an increase in beta-amyloid; a 2019 study added more to this emerging picture.

Tau is a standard chemical found in the brain; when the tau proteins clump together into tangles, they injure nearby tissue, causing cognitive decline. This tends to happen in areas of the brain linked to memory and then spreads throughout the brain in dementia. Sleep disruption causes a rapid build-up and spread of tau in the brain.

What is missing is any study that randomises people to either get enough good-quality sleep or have a bad night for years on end and then measures their brain function. This would prove getting enough sleep could prevent MCI and dementia. But prioritising adequate sleep is essential, especially around menopause when that can feel like a pipe dream.

Give up shift work

One prospective study of 3232 people found that doing shift work for 10 or more years takes a toll on your brain function. Ten years of shift work aged the brain an extra 6.5 years. The problem was not insufficient sleep, the study authors said: 'Rather, it seems likely that our findings reflect the disruption of the shift workers' circadian rhythms, which has been shown by other researchers to have an impact on brain structures involved in cognition and mental health over the lifespan.'

Their study did, however, find that the negative effects of shift work on the brain reversed when the shift work came to an end. But it took up to five years to achieve full recovery.

Exercise your brain

Lots of my patients tell me they do Sudoku to train their brains. Awesome! Lots of companies have been spruiking online games that promise eternal brain youth. Sadly, the evidence isn't great to support these pretty outrageous claims. Studies have shown that brain training can improve performance on the particular task that is being trained. In other words, we have evidence that doing Sudoku makes you better at doing Sudoku. However, the transfer of that benefit to a different cognitive domain isn't shown in studies. So if you enjoy particular online games or crosswords, then keep doing them. But let's not overplay what they're doing to ward off dementia.

But, before you give up and go back to watching *Married At First Sight* on loop, we *do* have evidence of the 'use it or lose it' concept for the brain. New exposure to what we call 'novel stimuli' seems to not only grow new neurons but also to create new 'connections' between neurons (called synapses). As experiences are repeated, these new neural pathways and connections are strengthened. Known as neuroplasticity, this process is probably best summarised by the phrase 'Neurons that fire together wire together'. The concept started when we discovered that rats with a more exciting and challenging environment had thicker brain cortices. It turns out that demanding mental tasks that require more complex brain wiring actually make humans grow more brain cells with more connections between them.

The latest evidence suggests that it is a *lifetime* of mentally stimulating and challenging activities that stands you in best stead. So start now! Enrol in a Spanish class, learn ballroom dancing, study poetry, read the papers and even learn to brush your teeth with your left hand (assuming you're right-handed). It's *the learning of new skills* that is the key, not just doing Sudoku over and over again.

Get a hearing aid (if you're deaf!)

We've known for a while that deafness increases your risk of MCI and dementia; probably by stopping you having proper social interactions, which then has a direct impact on your brain. Studies of getting your hearing fixed as a preventer of dementia haven't been done, but most experts agree we tend to under-recognise and under-treat hearing loss.

Chew gum

We've already noted the effect of chewing gum on mood, but how about its effect on your brainpower? Studies actually show that chewing gum is linked to higher productivity and fewer cognitive errors at work. But not improved memory. I have no explanation for this whatsoever; researchers claim they're going to do more study on what underpins the link. My late father would be horrified!

What medications and supplements are available?

HRT

It stands to reason that if low oestrogen contributes to a decline in brain function, then replacing it might help. Among younger women who are thrown into medical or surgical menopause, small clinical trials show that immediately starting HRT improves memory for verbal information, at least in the short term. But what about the rest of us? The International Menopause Society clearly states that starting HRT during the midlife period is associated with a reduced risk of Alzheimer's disease and dementia. This is based on several small studies. There are some issues with this advice, in my opinion. The largest trial of HRT specifically for prevention of cognitive decline involved 180 healthy postmenopausal women aged 45 to 55 years with already established cognitive symptoms. The women were randomised to placebo or a combined formulation of conjugated equine oestrogen and medroxyprogesterone acetate. This is the WHI combo, if you remember. After four months, there were no significant differences in memory or other cognitive measures between the women.

In another two slightly larger trials, the KEEPS trial (among women within three years from the onset of menopause) and the ELITE trial (within six years of menopause onset), HRT didn't yield any benefits for cognitive brainpower.

And then, in 2019, a Finnish study found that women who had taken HRT (any form) had a 10–20 per cent *higher* risk of developing Alzheimer's disease than women who hadn't been on HRT! Of the women with Alzheimer's disease, 18.6 per cent of women said they had used HRT at some stage. While only 17 per cent said they'd never taken it.

Well, that certainly set alarm bells ringing, although perhaps not in the way you'd think. Eager to prevent another WHI car crash, academics from all over the world raced to critique the paper. For example, academics pointed out, women who started taking HRT before the age of 60 did *not* have an increased risk of dementia unless they stayed on it for at least 10 years. Other experts pointed to the poor quality of memory of women in their eighties with Alzheimer's disease, which was used to retrospectively analyse who had taken HRT and who hadn't.

So where does that all leave you? No changes have been made to the International Menopause Society's recommendations that:

1. The reason for going on HRT is for the treatment of bothersome hot flushes or vasomotor symptoms.
2. HRT should not be used (solely) for the prevention or treatment of cognitive difficulties in women.
3. No clinical trial has yet specifically studied the long-term effects of HRT on cognitive function in women with moderate to severe vasomotor symptoms.
4. Available data from three randomised, placebo-controlled clinical trials provides reassurance that HRT initiated in the early postmenopausal years does not result in early adverse effects on cognitive function.

Testosterone supplements

The evidence just isn't in yet. The studies we have so far can be called, at worst, interesting and, at best, super exciting. If more studies are undertaken, we will be in a much better position to know whether these can help ward off or even reverse dementia.

L-carnitine

We discussed L-carnitine for weight loss in Chapter 7. It transports long-chain fatty acids into the mitochondria, the engines of our cells, so they can be burned to produce energy. It then turns around and removes the waste products that build up after the energy-burning process and removes them from the cell. Our bodies make some L-carnitine, and we get the rest from food — mainly animal products such as meat, dairy and eggs.

It is actually the decline in mitochondrial function that is thought to contribute to the aging process across the entire body. So researchers have been fascinated by the potential for L-carnitine to help stop age-related brain deterioration.

Here's what we know: the concentration of L-carnitine in tissues declines with age. And this decline contributes to the declining function of the mitochondrial membrane. Studies in elderly rats found supplementation with high doses of acetyl-L-carnitine and alpha-lipoic acid (which is an antioxidant) reduced their rate of mitochondrial decay. The supplemented little rats ran around their cages more, and performed better on memory tasks, than the rats on a placebo.

The studies in humans are a bit less exciting. A Cochrane collaboration meta-analysis of the grand total of two double-blind, placebo-controlled studies in humans (average age 21) concluded that supplements of acetyl-L-carnitine didn't do anything meaningful to improve functioning in the brain. Another review of people with established dementia found no evidence of benefit from L-carnitine for cognition, severity of dementia or functional ability.

It is well tolerated as a supplement. At very high doses (more than 3g per day), your digestion might suffer and there have been reports of a fishy body odour, but we generally wouldn't use that high a dose. One Gwyneth.

Vitamin E

Vitamin E (tocopherol) is a fat-soluble vitamin that is found naturally in foods such as vegetable oils, grains, meat, poultry, eggs, fruit, vegetables and wheatgerm oil. You can also get it as a supplement. Vitamin E might have an important role in preventing the breakdown (peroxidation) of the fatty acids found in cell membranes.

So, it is known as an antioxidant. But can it work to prevent dementia? Well, there is a *bit* of evidence. For example, in studies of around 1500mg a day of vitamin E (which is around 10 times the recommended daily requirement) in patients who already have Alzheimer's disease, some showed some improvement. They improved their ability to do what we call the 'activities of daily living' more than patients treated with placebo. In other studies, blood markers of oxidative stress fell after vitamin E supplementation. Studies in older women suggest that high doses of vitamin E (and other antioxidants) might be linked to lower risk of vascular dementia and better cognitive function. Might . . . But nothing definite. There's just not enough evidence of its overall long-term effect on cognitive impairment to justify doctors recommending vitamin E to our patients, according to a Cochrane review. (By the way, make sure you're not having more than 3000mg of vitamin E from supplements per day, especially if you have any cardiac or vascular problems. There's a link to increased risk of impaired clotting leading to a higher rate of strokes.) One Gwyneth.

Vitamin B (B6, B9, B12)

Vitamin B supplements are very popular and lots of people take them to improve their brainpower. Many forms of vitamin B supplements have been studied for their effect on cognition, including vitamin B6, vitamin B9 (folate) and B12 (cyanocobalamin).

Vitamin B deficiencies have been linked to cognitive impairment. This could be because high levels of a chemical called homocysteine in the blood are linked to a higher risk of dementia. And one of the most common causes of high homocysteine levels is B6, B9 or B12 deficiency. So, the theory was that if we top up the vitamin B, we could prevent the high homocysteine and prevent the dementia.

A study in Ireland found that 12 per cent of the elderly had B12 deficiency, while 15 per cent had B9 or folate deficiency. So supplementing deficient vitamins makes sense for brain health. But in terms of taking B vitamins as a general measure, without a deficiency, their popularity runs way ahead of the evidence. Sadly, systematic reviews of clinical (albeit small) trials of vitamin B supplements to prevent the progression of cognitive impairment have been pretty dismal. Scarily, in fact, some studies show that high doses of vitamin B might even increase depressive symptoms in patients with Alzheimer's disease. Two Gwyneths.

Vitamins A and C

Both vitamins A and C are antioxidants. Sadly, studies of using these supplements to prevent dementia have shown them not to work. One Gwyneth.

Vitamin D

We've known for years about the importance of vitamin D in protecting the health of the bones. It is actually made in the skin when it is exposed to sunshine. But for ardent sun avoiders, you can get smaller amounts directly from your diet (eggs and oily fish) or from supplements. It does *something* in the brain, too. Scientists have found vitamin D receptors in the cerebral cortex (which controls movement and cognitive function) as well as in the hippocampus (linked to cognitive function and memory).

Vitamin D might have nerve-preserving actions as well as anti-inflammatory, antioxidant and even anti-ischaemic (stroke-preventing) effects. One large Norwegian study found that people with extremely low blood levels of vitamin D were more than twice as likely as those with normal vitamin D levels to develop dementia. But the studies to say that taking vitamin D supplements (or even just spending a bit more time in the sun to raise your vitamin D levels naturally) will prevent dementia or even MCI have been disappointing. One Gwyneth.

Ginkgo biloba

Ginkgo biloba is one of *the most popular* supplements used for brain health, with the usual dose being 120–240mg per day. It comes from a particular Asian maidenhair tree; an extract of the leaves, which contain flavonoids and other 'magical' chemicals, is used in lots of Chinese medicines. Scientists have thought that ginkgo biloba might improve brain function by increasing blood supply by dilating blood vessels in the brain and reducing the number of damaging 'oxygen free radicals' that destabilise and kill cells.

Early studies got off to a promising start with some good results. But the more recent studies have been pretty disappointing, generally suggesting it does nothing for preventing dementia. There has been a major Cochrane review of ginkgo biloba for dementia prevention, which found mixed results. Three of the four more recent, larger, higher quality studies found no benefit over placebo, with the fourth study finding a massive benefit. The Cochrane authors found it to be pretty safe, but experts point out that it does interact with lots of common medicines. So run it by your GP or pharmacist before taking. One Gwyneth.

Coconut oil

I was never a fan of coconut oil. Not because of the taste, but the hype. When online Hollywood 'wellness' gurus start touting it, I instantly put on my sceptic's hat. But then I watched paediatrician Dr Mary Newport's TED talk about using coconut oil to treat her husband's devastating dementia, and I was floored by it. I went straight out and bought some for Daniel. After all, what did we have to lose? He earnestly tried — and kept it down once. Then he claimed he'd rather get dementia than have to eat spoons of this stuff every day! I rather like it — but is there any actual science behind it?

The claim is based on the theory that the brain cells of people with Alzheimer's disease are unable to use glucose to produce energy properly, and so the nerve cells 'starve'. Coconut oil was once scorned because it contains high levels of saturated fat, which we know contributes to heart diseases. It turns out the types of saturated fats in coconut oil are primarily medium-chain (MCFA) and some short-chain fatty acids. MCFAs are unique in that they are easily absorbed and metabolised by the liver, and are broken down immediately into ketones for use rather than being stored.

In Alzheimer's, there appears to be a pathological decrease in the brain's ability to use glucose. Some believe the ketones that are the breakdown products of the MCFAs in coconut oil may act as an alternative energy source for the brain. So that's the theory. Now for the science . . .

There aren't really any negative studies; there just aren't enough robust scientific studies to come down hard one way or the other. We might have some more details soon, as a study funded by the US National Institutes of Health is currently being carried out at the University of South Florida. In the meantime, experts still warn us to keep coconut-oil consumption to a small amount because we don't know its effect on cardiovascular health. One Gwyneth.

Ginseng

When I went on a trip to China, ginseng — the entire root — was in every pharmacy. Over there it is touted for all sorts of health benefits, with dementia prevention top among the claims. I wondered then, did the evidence stack up? Scientists believe that ginseng prevents the toxic build-up of the beta-amyloid protein that we believe causes dementia. Some studies have been done in very specific populations and have shown cognitive improvement in patients with Alzheimer's treated with 4.5–9g per day of Korean red ginseng. That's great, but in systematic reviews of these studies, the scientists have said we're not there yet. Different ginseng supplements at widely varying doses in these tiny studies mean that we can't make any firm conclusions either way. That seems a real shame, given the need and the popularity of the supplement. In any case, ginseng supplements seem to be very safe. Zero Gwyneths, because it's not terribly expensive.

Fish oil

Again, this is one of the most popular supplements for protecting brain function. It's been around only since the 1990s, when a bunch of studies were published showing various health benefits. There were reported benefits for cardiovascular diseases, various forms of arthritis, brain development and function, including mental illness and cognitive decline.

So what is it about fish oil that gives it magical properties? Fish oil has omega-3 fatty acids — also known as polyunsaturated fatty acids (PUFAs) — which are essential fatty acids that humans cannot synthesise efficiently from other substances. We need to get them either from our diet or from supplements. Within omega-3 fatty acids there are three different types of fatty acids: alpha-linolenic acid (ALA), eicosapentaenoic acid (EPA) and docosahexaenoic acid (DHA). ALA is found mainly in plant oils such as soy, flaxseed and canola. DHA and EPA are found in fish and seafood. Right now DHA is receiving most attention because it is essential for cognitive functioning throughout the life cycle, from conception and birth through to your death. DHA is the main long-chain polyunsaturated fatty acid present in the brain and it has a few specific functions. For example, it seems to increase the activity of certain enzymes in the membranes of the brain cells, enhance the receptors that sit on those membranes, and help with both the production and the function of neurotransmitters.

Scientists have found that progressively, as we get older, the concentration of DHA in the brain slowly declines, and this is more pronounced in older people with cognitive impairment. People suffering with Alzheimer's have 60–70 per cent less DHA in both blood and brain compared to people of the same age without dementia.

In animal studies, increasing the amount of DHA in the diet boosts neurotransmitter levels and reduces brain damage. In humans, prospective studies have shown that eating lots of oily fish seems to protect us against developing Alzheimer's disease. In the enormous and long-lasting Framingham study in the US, low levels of DHA were associated with an increased risk for the development of dementia.

If you like eating fish and seafood, you're in luck! One study from 2016 showed that eating just one meal a week of fish or seafood for a year was linked to less decline in certain types of memory and mental processing speed.

There have been some great results from randomised, double-blind, placebo-controlled clinical trials of fish-oil supplements with high concentrations of DHA and EPA. In the MIDAS study, 485 patients with MCI were given a supplement of 900mg per day of DHA or placebo for six months. In this study significant improvements in learning and memory were seen in those taking DHA but not the placebo. DHA has also been studied in combination with EPA. In a prospective study, a combination of DHA and EPA was associated with improvement in the cognitive function of patients with MCI, but also in patients who already had Alzheimer's disease. They also showed improved short-term memory in patients with MCI. This is great news, but the studies are so small . . . As in, less than 20 patients per study.

These studies have been small, of poor quality and often done in people with established dementia, which has a pretty terrible prognosis anyway. The Cochrane review of omega-3 fatty acids for the prevention of dementia and cognitive impairment gave a conclusion that fell well short of a full recommendation. Apart from the usual step of calling for bigger and better studies, the authors basically said that, based on the evidence we have so far, it wasn't much better than placebo.

I think that raising your blood levels of omega-3 fats is worth a shot. The evidence for having fish and seafood in the diet is the most compelling. But if you hate seafood, you can try a supplement. Side effects of the supplements can be pretty annoying — a nasty taste in the mouth, bad breath, heartburn, stomach ache, diarrhoea, headaches and body odour. The dose? A bit of a guess right now: doses in studies range from 250mg to 1800mg DHA per day.

The American Food and Drug Administration says we should take no more than 3g per day of EPA and DHA combined. This includes up to 2g per day from dietary supplements. Higher doses could cause bleeding problems and possibly even reduce immune system function. Zero Gwyneths, as long as you don't take too much!

THE SHARPEST TOOL IN THE SHED

THE BOTTOM LINE

Brain aging is inevitable. Menopause seems to make it worse.

The best methods we have right now to prevent dementia are exercise, diet and socialising.

When it comes to HRT and testosterone — don't bank on them helping your brain.

Some supplements might play a role, but the evidence is a bit thin still.

CHAPTER 9

MAKE ME LOOK LIKE HELEN MIRREN

This chapter won't be for everyone. It might even offend some women; if that's you, please accept my sincerest apologies. Not every woman puts a huge emphasis on her looks; many don't care a jot. And I agree that your health — physical, mental and spiritual — trumps the size of your bottom or the colour of your hair. If you honestly don't care about your appearance one way or the other, please feel free to skip this chapter. It will not diminish your chances of having a positive menopause experience one little bit.

But more women care than I had ever realised, and I'm going to share a couple of stories to explain how I've developed a massive passion for this area. I've been a 'TV doctor' for over 10 years now; my regular gig is as the Channel 7 *Sunrise* GP. *Sunrise* is the top-rating breakfast TV show in Australia, and I'm also the host of *Embarrassing Bodies Down Under* and *Medicine or Myth?* When I started TV work, I was in my early forties and I noticed a certain pattern: every time we did a *Sunrise* segment on 'what really works in anti-aging skin care', I would speak about the evidence for specific ingredients we should look for in our skin care, rather than spruiking any particular products. But as soon as the segment finished, I would be inundated with questions — often up to 300 emails asking:

'So what products should I be using?' And my GP patients would also, after a pap test or heart check, casually slip in: 'So, what moisturiser do you recommend?'

It should be easy enough to find a good range of products to suggest, I thought. I'll look into it!

My personal focus at this stage was looking OK on TV. I've spent my entire life hating my skin. I have what is called 'combination skin', which means I spent my teenage years with an oil slick in my T zone and a face like a pizza. I continued to get acne breakouts throughout my pregnancies and well into my forties. And yet, my skin is also really dry and sensitive, and I react to many skin products. So, my poor face can have both zits and dry, red, scaly patches simultaneously. And now I was being caked in heavy foundation to film TV segments multiple times a week. My skin was not getting any better.

Despite searching, I'd never found my skincare nirvana. Products that dried out my zits would burn and sting, leaving my skin red and dry. Products that got rid of my flaky skin came with a side order of pimples. Until that time, I had never factored aging into my skincare search. But the more I researched skin care for aging, downloading studies from the National Library of Medicine, the more I saw the synergies between the actives that worked for aging and the actives that work for acne. Plus, when I looked in the mirror, I couldn't deny that in my forties I was developing all the signs of aging: fine lines, wrinkles, pigmentation.

So, armed with a new-found enthusiasm for skincare products in the anti-aging space, I embarked on a serious product search. Based only on science. And I found . . . nothing. I found products that were close — often very close — but not quite there. I found products that were nowhere near close — and everything in-between. But I couldn't find even one serum or cream I wanted to use, let alone recommend to our *Sunrise* viewers. This, despite sciency-looking symbols, and claims of being 'scientifically proven' or 'dermatologically tested'. So much noise, and all of it baseless hype! And this made me furious. Pseudoscience for financial gain is annoying enough, but women were forking out bucketloads of cash for products that were making entirely baseless claims. It felt incredibly unjust.

I copied and pasted a series of email replies to our viewers. 'I am searching for the ultimate products and, when I find them, I'll email you back.' But I never did email them back. Because the promised products just didn't exist. I approached a local compounding pharmacist, asking him whether I could write a prescription for an evidence-based vitamin C preparation. That would be L-ascorbic acid in a 10 per cent concentration, with a pH below 3.5 and in a water-in-oil emulsion, as per the peer-reviewed studies. He explained why he couldn't do it. For a start, L-ascorbic acid is highly unstable and is broken down by both air and light. So it needs to be handled in a dark room using infra-red glasses. The pharmacy back room was out of the question! Plus, it really needed to be stored in an airless bottle (with a pump that doesn't allow air to mix with the remaining ingredients in the bottle). And it needed to be stored in a light-repellent container, which ruled out droppers and glass bottles. And yet, so many products I had looked at were in droppers! Or it had to be used inside a week. Why was this so hard?

One night, over dinner with Daniel, I had a rant about the entire skincare industry. I lamented that, despite enormous claims, the industry seems to be entirely based on nice smells and nice feel, rather than on the science that is easily and widely available in scientific literature. You only had to search the National Library of Medicine to see the evidence — it was all there! This was exploitation of women! And laziness! Plus a missed market opportunity. Daniel casually said: 'Why don't you make your own skincare range then? How hard could it be?'

'I just don't have the time,' I said, sadly.

That was the start of our skincare journey. Daniel, who was working in property finance, would come home at night and, after the kids went to bed, we'd head to our pet project. We created a spreadsheet, using the available published data, to create our 'wish list' in terms of a skincare range. We researched formulations, pH, carrier systems, preservatives, sunscreens . . . everything. Then, between meetings with investors, Daniel met with formulation chemists and regulators, emailed ingredient manufacturers in the US and Europe, and met manufacturers. David, our second oldest, had gone backpacking for six months, so Daniel took over his room.

There he amassed thousands of bottles that he checked for quality and dispensing.

I can't tell you how or when this side project graduated from absorbing interest to compelling occupation. But by the time David got home from overseas and wanted his room back, we were both all in. There were so many hurdles. One of our most important ingredients was almost impossible to procure; we needed a special licence to import it, which was not easy to get. We had to transport it from a factory in Europe to a manufacturer in Sydney at -20 degrees Celsius. Without breaking the cold chain. We ordered bottles that failed and we had to throw away a bunch of products after bottling. Goods valued at the price of a small car went into the tip, and we both took on extra work in our day jobs to recover the lost money. But, after a year, we had it: an evidence-based skincare range that was simple (only six products initially) and entirely faithful to the published, peer-reviewed studies.

We started by partnering with plastic surgeons and dermatologists across Australia, creating private-label ranges for them. The reason we took that route was pretty simple: we had no money to spend on marketing and advertising. And to cut through in the world of skincare hype, you need to shout loudly and spend big. But dermatologists and plastic surgeons were much more aware of the evidence and they saw what we had created for what it was. We didn't necessarily win over the commercially ambitious doctors, but the science nerds all quickly came onboard.

These early adopters of evidence-based skin care were more than just customers: they were partners and collaborators. They helped develop the next few products with us and refine the existing ones. And eventually Daniel and I felt ready to roll out our little brand, ESK (for Evidence Skin care).

I look at pictures of myself from six years ago, before we came up with our skincare range, and the difference in my skin is amazing. I look 10 years younger now. In my fifties, I have finally beaten the breakouts, even at 'that time of the month'. I also have less pigmentation, fine lines and wrinkles. My pores are smaller and my skin feels so smooth. I can't believe I ever had rough, flaky crocodile skin! That is the feedback we get from our customers, too, and it is what studies tell us should happen. I had Botox once in 2012: I haven't needed it since. If my face is still on TV in ten years I might do it again, but luckily, for now, I just don't need it.

I share this story to explain how a fierce feminist became passionate about having the option to choose to look your best. It's not saving lives, but in a world of rampant consumerism and marketing, it gives our customers, and us, such great joy. So, if you want this skincare information, you should be able to get it without having to wade through mucky marketing messages.

What's happening to my face and skin as I age?

Lots of changes happen to the actual shape of your face as you get older. Firstly, many of your facial bones become thinner and flatter in places. For example, your eye sockets lose some of their bone mass so your eyes look more sunken; your muscles and ligaments, which underpin the skin, shrink and loosen; you lose fat from under the skin so your blood vessels seem more prominent. And some of what are known as 'fat pads' actually move (downwards — thanks, gravity!). All of these factors contribute to an older facial appearance before we even look at what happens to your skin.

The skin is made up of three layers, each with certain functions:

- Epidermis
- Dermis
- Subcutaneous fat layer (hypodermis)

Epidermis

The whole point of skin is protection against water loss from the body and the prevention of substances and germs penetrating into the body. This is what we call the 'skin barrier function' and it is mainly performed by the epidermis. The epidermis is the thin outer layer of the skin. It consists of four types of cells:

Squamous cells make up the outermost layer of the skin, the stratum corneum. Skin cells from this layer are continuously being shed.

Basal cells are found just under the squamous cells, at the base of the epidermis. They migrate upwards and become squamous cells, eventually being shed.

Melanocytes are found throughout the epidermis. They make your pigment or melanin (melanin's role is to protect your skin from ultraviolet radiation).

Langerhans cells are part of the immune system and help the epidermis fight attempted invasion from bacteria, fungi and viruses, as well as chemical injuries.

Dermis

The dermis is the middle layer of the skin and is 20 to 30 times thicker than the epidermis. The dermis consists of a whole variety of cells and structures, including your blood and lymphatic vessels, nerves, hair follicles, sweat glands, collagen bundles (the scaffolding of the skin that helps keep its shape, strength and integrity), elastin (part of that scaffolding network, too), fibroblasts to make the collagen, and hyaluronic acid, nerves and sebaceous glands that make oil.

Subcutaneous fat layer

The subcutaneous fat is the deepest layer of skin. It not only contains fat cells, but also a lot of collagen, and it acts as your body's insulator, as well as its shock absorber. Its layers are not smooth and even, rather they're almost wavy in appearance. The waviness seems to protect your skin from injuries, as well as more firmly anchoring the layers of the skin together. This waviness is a key feature, and the layers even out as you get older.

Clinical Associate Professor Saxon Smith is a dermatologist at The University of Sydney. I spoke to him about menopause and skin, and he pointed out that, as well as increasing wrinkles and sagging skin, losing subcutaneous fat also leads to easy bruising. It also means the blood vessels become more prominent and you look blotchier as a result. Gravitational drop can mean a thinner face with fat accumulating around the jowls, usually made worse by the disappearance of your cheekbones. Yes, your bones actually start to ebb away around your eyes, making the hollows of your eyes more pronounced.

The role of hormones in skin

It's hard to tease out how many of the changes in your skin are due to age and how many to menopause. Certainly anecdotally, women tell me menopause ushers in some pretty big negative changes.

In menopause, skin quickly loses collagen, which thins it and weakens its structure. Studies show that a woman's skin loses about 30 per cent of its collagen within the first five years of menopause. After that, we continue to lose a further 2 per cent every year for the next 20 years. OMG! The effect? Well, it's not good news. Our skin loses its firmness and starts to sag. Permanent lines develop from the tip of the nose to the corners of the mouth. Wrinkles become more prominent. You might see bags under your eyes. Your pores can look larger as a direct result of a lack of skin firmness. Big pores make your skin look and feel rougher and less even.

The pH of your skin becomes significantly elevated in your first years of menopause (age 50 to 60). This sees the microbiome of the skin, or the bacteria that live happily on your skin, alter significantly. The clinical significance of this is an emerging field. But dermatologists think these changes might contribute to skin aging.

It's not just about menopause, though. Sun exposure (which accumulates over a lifetime) and, to a lesser extent, other pollutants can make aging changes worse. This is called 'extrinsic aging'.

'Intrinsic aging' is an unpreventable process, and affects the skin in the same way it affects all our internal organs. Lucky genes can, to some degree, help reduce the dramatic effects of 'intrinsic aging'.

Aging skin

Youthful skin retains its strength, resilience and flexibility because of its high content of water. Photo aging (as a result of exposure to the sun's UVA rays) and just the normal process of aging cause loss of moisture. The key molecule involved in skin moisture is hyaluronic acid (HA), which has a fascinating unique ability to hold and retain water in the skin. It makes up a large part of the 'extracellular matrix' — the spongy network that, with collagen, forms the scaffolding and structure in which your cells sit. HA drops off dramatically, especially from the epidermis, as skin starts to age.

In addition, sebum, your skin's natural oil, continues to drop over the course of your lifetime. In total you'll see around a 60 per cent fall from peak levels. This means your skin will become naturally drier.

In young healthy skin, collagen is continuously turned over. It is broken down by enzymes called metalloproteinases and then resynthesised by fibroblasts. The brand new, long strands of collagen give your skin its strength and flexibility. As your skin ages, your fibroblasts have a reduced capacity to divide and less ability to produce collagen. Then, UV radiation makes your skin produce *more* metalloproteinases, which shifts the skin's balance towards collagen breakdown. The collagen that remains can clump together, giving the skin a 'cobblestoned' appearance.

Less new collagen means less scaffolding, which means thinner skin, skin sagging and the appearance of larger pores, fine lines and wrinkles. More collagen is like the Holy Grail of skin care!

Aging is also inevitably associated with a decrease in elastin. The elastin you do retain grows more calcified and broken down. This all means the skin gets stiffer.

The epidermis becomes thinner. The most marked evidence of this thinning is seen on the face, neck, upper part of the chest and the backs of the hands and forearms. Epidermal thinning continues with a loss of around 6.4 per cent per decade on average. Your subcutaneous fat levels will reduce by as much as a 65 per cent. Melanocytes start to die off, decreasing at a rate of 8 to 20 per cent per decade. The result? Uneven pigmentation in elderly skin.

Can sunscreen help prevent my skin from aging?

Hands down the biggest source of aging that you can actually prevent is sun exposure. Approximately 80 per cent of facial-skin aging is attributed to UV exposure! The sun emits ultraviolet radiation (UV), and sunscreens (called broad-spectrum sunscreens) target UVA and UVB rays. As a rough rule of thumb, you see this as 'B for burning'. The short-wavelength UVB rays will be most fierce between 11am and 3pm in the middle of summer and are the most damaging when it comes to skin cancers such as melanoma. Think of the long-wavelength UVA rays as 'A for aging' (and tanning). They make up 95 per cent of UV radiation that reaches earth from the sun. Most photo-aging happens as a result of exposure to UVA rays, which are present across the day from sunrise to sunset, throughout the year. We now know they do also contribute to skin cancer, but not nearly as much as UVB rays.

If you care about sun-related aging, you need sunscreen from sunrise to sunset right through the year. It can go under your makeup, but it doesn't matter that you're only seeing sunlight on your way to and from work: it all adds up.

How to choose an everyday sunscreen

SPF is one of the most poorly understood concepts there is. SPF is a measure of UVB protection only, and tells you nothing about UVA protection. SPF does not mean the *amount* of protection per se; rather, it indicates how *long* it will take for UVB rays to burn your skin when you're using a given sunscreen, compared to how long skin *would have taken* to burn without the sunscreen on. So, someone using an SPF 15 sunscreen will take 15 times longer to burn than when they have no sunscreen on. An SPF 15 sunscreen screens 93 per cent of the sun's UVB rays; SPF 30 protects against 97 per cent; and SPF 50, 98 per cent. The Skin Cancer Foundation in the US recommends you use a sunscreen of SPF 15 or higher, but that for more extended or intense sun exposure (going to the beach or taking a long hike), you use SPF 30 or higher.

How do you know what UVA filters are in the sunscreen? That is less well regulated. Broad spectrum or multi spectrum indicates both UVA and UVB filters are in the sunscreen. But specific UVA-filtering ingredients include avobenzone, ecamsule, oxybenzone, titanium dioxide and zinc oxide. The first three are chemical sunscreens, while the last two are what we call 'physical sunscreens' (also sometimes called mineral sunscreens).

While chemical sunscreens are far more common than physical sunscreens, here are the reasons I always choose physical sunscreens:

- They block both UVA and UVB rays (all physical sunscreens are broad spectrum and block the UVA rays rather than absorbing and keeping them away from your skin cells, as chemical sunscreens do). However, because zinc oxide is a superior UVA filter to titanium dioxide, I would always choose a zinc-based product over titanium-based.

- They start working as soon as you put them on (you have to wait for 20 minutes for chemical sunscreens to start working).

- They cause less irritation than chemical sunscreens, so are a good choice for sensitive skin.

- Both titanium dioxide and zinc oxide are 'non comedogenic', so don't cause acne breakouts. Mind you, the other ingredients they're mixed with can!

- Physical sunscreens can limit acne rosacea and redness, as they block the heat from UVA rays from the skin (rather than absorbing both the UVA and UVB and converting that energy to heat, as chemical sunscreens do).

The downside of physical sunscreens is that they tend to feel pore-cloggingly thick and gooey on your face, as well as leaving a ghostly white tinge to your skin. This means many women won't use them, especially not every day. Let me explain that it's all about the way they're formulated. Our ESK sunscreen formulation chemist nearly tore her hair out trying to get us a product we were happy with. It took no less than 23 attempts to get Zinc Shade, our ESK zinc oxide day cream formulation. Zinc Shade sits nicely with or without make-up on top and doesn't look or feel white or thick at all.

A cautionary note about oxybenzone. The Environmental Working Group (a not-for-profit organisation that assesses ingredients and products for their risk of harm) scores this at 8 — a very high risk of hazard. (Anything rated 6 or over is hazardous.) As well as an ability to cause allergic skin reactions, oxybenzone also appears to be a weak oestrogen. This mightn't be an issue for women around menopause age, but the US Center for Disease Control analysed American children and found that adolescent boys with higher oxybenzone measurements had significantly lower total testosterone levels. For the sake of the people around you, I'd urge you not to use products containing oxybenzone. Another one to avoid is octinoxate (also called octylmethoxycinnamate), which has a rating of 6.

My three sunscreen tips:

1. It's never too late to start using sunscreen, even if you have well-developed sun damage on your skin.
2. Use enough! It needs to be evenly distributed all over your skin to do its job. You can't miss any bits!
3. Use it not only on your face but also on your neck and 'décolletage'. I also put it on the backs of my hands every day.

How should I clean my skin?

There are three reasons we clean our skin, particularly the skin on our faces:

1. Cosmetic: getting the grime, make-up, dead skin cells and grease off our face makes it look nicer. It's something we've been doing for a long time, with the first recorded soaps dating back 4000 years.
2. As a precursor to skin care: removing the layer of dirt from your skin allows skincare products to penetrate the skin and do their work better.
3. For managing breakouts, if you get them. A build-up of dirt on the skin can block your pores and increase the likelihood of acne.

Cleaning with soap can be a disaster, especially for sensitive facial skin and the thinner, drier skin of menopause. Soaps are made up of long-chain fatty acids combined with alkaline salts, and have a pH between 9 and 10, while the skin's natural pH sits at around 5. Surfactants in soap break down the bond between fats, which allows them to be washed away. So it's not surprising that soap increases the pH of the skin and decreases the skin's fat content, which dries it out. A higher pH alone leads to dryness, compromising the skin's barrier function and reducing flexibility.

Some ingredients in soap can do more harm than good. Some surfactants are too good at their job and can damage the skin. Aggressive surfactants (such as common soap ingredient sodium laurel sulphate) can break down some of the fats and proteins that form part of the protective outer layer of the skin, reducing the skin's ability to retain moisture, making it drier and increasing its sensitivity. Gentler alternatives include coco glucoside, sodium lauryl methyl isethionate and lauryl glucoside. Hence choosing a soap-free cleanser is important at any stage, but especially around menopause.

When you are buying a cleanser, bear in mind that it can't do much more than cleanse. I know that sounds obvious, but if you're spending $100 on a cleanser, you're probably hoping for some miracle property. I can tell you now that you'll be disappointed. A cleanser is usually in contact with your skin for a limited time and any active ingredient in it is usually washed off before it can be absorbed. If a cleanser does instruct you to leave it on the skin for a few minutes, this will be to allow an ingredient time to act — I'm thinking specifically of alphahydroxy acids and salicylic acid for the management of acne.

What can I put on my skin to combat aging?

When it comes to ingredients that can help with skin aging, there are hundreds that are marketed as being 'the best' or just plain old 'miraculous'. I will only cover those that have the best evidence. No miracles here — just ingredients that we know work.

Vitamin A, the ultimate anti-aging superstar

Listen here, sisters, if you aren't using vitamin A in your skincare regime, you're missing out. In prescription form it is the *best-studied and most effective* ingredient for anti-aging (it also has evidence for management of acne and rosacea).

Our bodies can't create vitamin A. But we get it through our diet, either as beta-carotene or retinyl palmitate. It is then converted in the skin to retinol, then converted again to retinal and finally to retinoic acid. That process is critically important. Retinoic acid (which you can get on prescription from your doctor *right now*) is where the magic happens. We have several receptors in our skin that specifically respond to retinoic acid. When triggered, these receptors cause a cascade of events that result in skin renewal. We're talking thicker, more elastic, more youthful-looking skin, with fewer wrinkles, fine lines, roughness, freckles and pigmentation. Sound good?

That's the simple part. Unfortunately, the prescription form (the best-studied form) is often irritating and drying. In my practice, I do prescribe it frequently for acne but I often find that my patients just can't push through the initial irritation and they stop using it.

In looking for effective but better-tolerated versions of vitamin A, manufacturers have turned to other forms, in the hope of getting the results without the irritation. You might see 'retinyl palmitate', 'retinyl glucoside', 'retinyl propionate', 'retinol' or 'retinal' listed as ingredients on the label. They are all forms of vitamin A. But they don't all have the same evidence, or effectiveness. While retinol and retinyl palmitate are the most common forms of vitamin A used in skin care, it is actually retinal that has the best evidence and is the least irritating form. Retinol is still two steps away from becoming the active form, retinoic acid. That means a lot of it needs to be used to get a reasonable dose of retinoic acid in the skin, and that high dose of retinol can be irritating. Some people don't have sufficient enzyme levels in the skin to convert the retinol to retinal, so it is also less effective.

And that (together with not being able to find many evidence-based forms of vitamin C) is why I started ESK. We could find only a handful of brands that used retinal and they were either super expensive, very hard to get (only through a few doctors' practices) or packaged up with preservatives, stabilisers and perfumes that had dodgy safety ratings.

And it's also what makes our Ultimate A and Ultimate A+ our hero products. With a retinal concentration of 0.06 per cent (for anti-aging and rosacea), Ultimate A is our go-to anti-aging night cream. And at 0.1 per cent concentration, the Ultimate A+ is used for acne or oilier and thicker skin (such as that of men, for example).

Vitamin C, an anti-aging essential

Why is this little vitamin such a staple of cosmeceutical anti-aging skin care? For a start, when vitamin C is applied to the skin, it acts as an antioxidant — it reduces and reverses pigmentation, wrinkles, fine lines and skin roughness, and protects from UV radiation. It also promotes collagen growth.

Best known as the vitamin needed to protect from scurvy, vitamin C (L-ascorbic acid) is a naturally occurring antioxidant contained in most fruits and vegetables. Vitamin C helps repair damaged and worn-out tissues by scavenging free radicals that are formed when we are exposed to pollutants such as radiation and cigarette smoke. Over time, the build-up of free radicals is largely responsible for the aging process — they are also thought to play a role in cancer, as well as a number of chronic conditions including heart disease and arthritis.

The biggest problem with vitamin C in skin care is that, as a chemical, it is water soluble and easily oxidised. This makes it difficult to formulate in a stable and effective form because water is needed to dissolve the vitamin C, but the water oxidises it! As the skin is good at keeping out water-soluble particles, it makes it difficult to get the vitamin C to penetrate the skin. Both of these problems can be overcome to some degree by formulating an L-ascorbic acid product at a pH of 3.5 or less. Or by formulating the vitamin C in a base that has no water (such as oil or silicone). Regardless of how you do it, there is a small but increased risk of skin irritation.

As a result, there are a number of different, more stable, forms of vitamin C that are used in skin care, in the hope that they will have the effect of vitamin C without the formulation difficulties. On a label you can spot these ingredients as the ones that have 'ascorbate' or 'ascorbyl' in their name. The problem with these ingredients is that, while manufacturers refer to them as vitamin C, their antioxidant abilities are much lower than L-ascorbic acid. Vitamin C (to be specific, L-ascorbic acid) was one of the main reasons I started ESK. It's an ingredient with good evidence of great anti-aging properties, but almost impossible to find in an evidence-based form. When I was trying to answer viewer emails about the best skin care,

I found lots of products claiming to contain 'vitamin C'. But they pretty much all used the non-evidence-based forms (yet the creative claims that were attached to many of those products were beyond belief).

ESK's Reverse C Serum contains L-ascorbic acid at 10 per cent concentration — the most common concentration in published studies in peer-reviewed journals. Studies also suggest that concentrations higher than 20 per cent will be ineffective and needlessly increase irritation. ESK's Reverse C Serum is one of my favourite products — it leaves my skin feeling hydrated all day and is great under my make-up. If you're looking for a vitamin C product, here are the things I would recommend looking for:

1. Look for L-ascorbic acid in the ingredient list.
2. The product should be clear or pale yellow. Oxidised ('off') vitamin C turns dark yellow, brown or orange. Beware of products that are dyed those colours . . . what are they hiding?
3. If the first ingredient listed is water, the product will not be stable and will go off.
4. The first ingredient listed should be an oil (or silicone).
5. If there are too many ingredients on the list, it is almost certain that one of them will oxidise the L-ascorbic acid and it will go off.

Vitamin B3, a great skincare all-rounder

Vitamin B3, or niacinamide, is one of the newer arrivals on the 'evidence-based' skincare ingredients list. And while most of the ingredients on that list are more than just 'one trick ponies', this one in particular has an impressive repertoire. It is used for anti-aging, management of some common skin disorders, managing acne and reducing the risk of non-melanoma skin cancer. Not only that, but it is well tolerated and very rarely causes reactions. However, it does come with some warnings, not all of which are heeded by everyone in the skincare industry.

We all get vitamin B3 from foods, mainly from meat, poultry and fish, but also from peanuts, brown rice and seeds, and to a lesser degree milk, bananas and tomatoes. More than 400 enzymes in the body need vitamin B3 to work, making it the vitamin most used in enzyme-based activity. Some of its main jobs are to assist in converting the energy stored in carbohydrates, fats and proteins into a form that can be used by our cells; to make sure that our genes remain 'healthy' (don't undergo inappropriate changes); and to make sure that our cells can protect themselves from oxidative stress.

Some of the first articles describing niacinamide's potential were published in 2002. It's not often that I would say this, but hats off to Procter & Gamble. They sponsored the first set of studies on vitamin B3, looking at its ability to reduce hyperpigmentation, sallowness (yellowing) and wrinkles. When it comes to evidence, industry sponsorship of a study isn't disqualifying but it does need to be taken with a pinch of salt. So, when these studies were followed by others, many of which were independently conducted, particularly looking at the role of vitamin B3 in preventing acne, as a moisturiser and for use in various skin conditions, the evidence for vitamin B3 and our confidence to use it in skincare formulations improved.

Niacinamide can help with a number of the common signs of skin aging, particularly depigmentation and management of age spots. As we get older, sun-induced age spots become the most obvious and observable indicator of skin aging. And, while we know that UV exposure causes age spots, we aren't exactly sure how they happen. While hyperpigmentation and age spots are notoriously difficult to treat, niacinamide does have some good evidence for these and the management of sallowness, wrinkles and skin elasticity.

In addition to its anti-aging benefits, vitamin B3 has anti-inflammatory properties and has been shown to improve the skin-barrier function. As a result, it also useful in managing several inflammatory skin conditions, including rosacea, eczema and psoriasis. And there's even more . . .

Due to its anti-inflammatory effects and its ability to regulate the skin's natural oil production, vitamin B3 is a good ingredient to use in managing acne. And, given that acne and rosacea are often hard to tell apart, that makes vitamin B3 one of the few ingredients that can help with both (and not irritate either). Last but not least, vitamin B3 is increasingly being recognised for reducing the risk of non-melanoma skin cancer, the most common form of cancer in Australia.

A word of caution about vitamin B3

A number of manufacturers have used increasingly higher concentrations of active ingredients in their skincare products in the mistaken belief that 'more is more'. And, particularly because it is so well tolerated, this happens with vitamin B3, where I've seen concentrations as high as 10 per cent. That's just not backed by evidence. The published studies of niacinamide in skin care used concentrations between 2.5 and 5 per cent. There is no good data on either effectiveness or side effects such as skin sensitivity for doses higher than that. And we know that ingesting high levels of vitamin B3 can lead to liver problems. We have used 4 per cent vitamin B3 in our Ultimate A and Ultimate A+ ESK night creams, 5 per cent in our Enlighten depigmentation cream, and 5 per cent in both our B Quenched and B Calm moisturisers for sensitive skin.

Exfoliators, the path to smoother skin

The idea behind exfoliation is to remove old, rough, dead skin cells, leaving the fresher, younger-looking, newer epidermal cells at the surface. When I was at the peak of my teenage acne, Mum took me to David Jones for some help. The lady behind the counter told her I needed to dry out my greasy skin, so Mum bought me a toner and a special soap. And I needed to rub my face daily with a face washer to exfoliate, and to use a scrub. From memory it had ground up apricot seeds in it. It smelled really nice. My skin got worse. Medically trained adult me is aghast at the awful information we were given in 1980. Apart from soap being just wrong (see below), toners in those days were alcohol-based, so stripped the water and fat from the skin cells, inflaming them and making my cells produce more oil to compensate. And, in terms of exfoliation, the face washer and scrubs did indeed exfoliate, but in a rough way that was again pro-inflammatory and would make my sensitive skin redder, drier in patches and make my acne worse.

These days, experts do still recommend exfoliation, but we do it with gentle chemicals. Alpha hydroxy acids (AHAs), or fruit acids as they are sometimes called, have probably been used in skin care longer than any other cosmeceutical ingredient. Legend has it that Cleopatra bathed in milk for her complexion. If that's right, it would make lactic acid (the alpha hydroxy acid from sour milk) our longest-used cosmeceutical, with a pedigree of over 2000 years. And yet, of the commonly used cosmeceuticals, AHAs have some of the sparsest evidence.

AHAs include ingredients such as glycolic acid, lactic acid, mandelic acid, malic acid and citric acid. (I've listed those in decreasing order of irritation.) The majority of studies have looked at glycolic and lactic acids, which have been shown to help in managing acne. And, at higher concentrations, they work pretty well for aging skin, too; they have been shown to increase collagen, reduce wrinkles and decrease pigmentation. Glycolic acid is also beneficial in helping other ingredients, particularly retinal, to work more effectively.

Having said all of that, as concentrations of AHAs increase in a product, the pH decreases (becomes more acidic) and irritation really starts to increase. Chemists reduce that irritation by adding buffers that simply increase the pH. The problem is that buffering the AHAs reduces their effectiveness, and the most commonly used buffering ingredient, sodium hydroxide, can itself be irritating to the skin. Another issue we discovered fairly recently is that using AHAs in higher concentrations brings a risk of hyperpigmentation for people with darker skin. AHAs also increase sun sensitivity, so you need to be more diligent with sunscreen.

So, how do you get the benefits of exfoliation from your AHA cosmeceuticals without the downside? We chose to formulate ESK's Smooth Serum with 3 per cent glycolic acid and 1 per cent lactic acid for use at night (under Ultimate A). At that concentration, it does a great job exfoliating for smoother skin, helps with the effectiveness of retinal (in Ultimate A night cream), is well tolerated on most skin, and does not need to be buffered. But not always . . . Some of us just have super-sensitive skin, especially those with rosacea, or just menopause-related skin sensitivity. If my skin is having a 'moment', I take a couple of days rest from putting Smooth Serum on my neck (for some reason that's my sensitive spot), then when I go back to it, it leaves my skin feeling smooth and soft.

Can I do anything about age spots?

We have a lot of ESK customers looking for help with pigmentation such as age or sun spots (solar lentigines). And it is small wonder a trial conducted in 2013 concluded that age spots, rather than wrinkles or fine lines, are the feature that visibly ages us most. So, if you want to address the signs of aging, this is a good place to start.

While we know that age spots are caused by repeated sun exposure, we still aren't exactly sure how that process works. Our current understanding is that, over time, UV exposure affects some of the genes in the skin with two main outcomes. Firstly, one of the skin layers forms deep ridges, which trap melanin (the pigment in skin), leading to a build-up. Secondly, there is an actual increased production of melanin. Hey presto — age spots appear. Before we begin to look at managing them, it's important to know that if you get age spots, you are at a higher risk of getting skin cancer and you should be getting regular skin checks.

Treating hyperpigmentation can be difficult and results are not guaranteed. So, now that I have lowered your expectations, let's look at what can be done. The most important factor in managing age spots is broad-spectrum sunscreen — it will reduce the risk of getting them in the first place, and reduce the risk of reoccurrence after treatment. Without using sunscreen, it is unlikely that any treatment will be effective.

For people with darker natural skin colour (Fitzpatrick skin types IV to VI), some of the most effective or aggressive treatments can result in hypo (too little) or hyper (too much) pigmentation. If you think that's you, I recommend a visit to a qualified skin doctor as a first step.

I'll deal with physical treatments such as dermabrasion, laser and peels later in the chapter. Let's discuss skin creams first, because, regardless of whether you use a topical treatment as a first-line treatment, or some other device-based treatment, you'll need active skin care for a maintenance regime at least.

Ingredients that can be used to manage age spots are divided into three groups by mechanism of activity. Using ingredients from different groups at the same time has a synergistic effect and will get you better results. So go for a product with a few different pigmentation ingredients or a few single ingredient products together to manage hyperpigmentation.

The first group of ingredients controls tyrosinase, which is one of the enzymes involved in making melanin. Most research has been done on tyrosinase inhibitors, which is believed to be the way to get the best results. Hydroquinone is the best known and has the best evidence to support it; however, there are significant and growing concerns about its side effects and safety, which have led to its being banned in a number of countries including Japan, the EU and South Africa (in concentrations of above 2 per cent). A planned ban by the American FDA is currently under review due to industry pressure. There are four other ingredients in this group — kojic acid, azelaic acid, arbutin and 4-n-butylresorcinol. So far, the evidence suggests that 4-n-butylresorcinol, while the least known of the ingredients, has the best combination of safety and effectiveness.

The second group of ingredients interferes with a key step in the creation of skin pigment, which involves the transfer of melanin from the melanocyte, where it is made, to the superficial skin cell called the keratinocyte. Niacinamide (vitamin B3) is one of the best-known ingredients in this group and has good evidence for pigmentation reduction.

The third group is the antioxidants. Among other things, they reduce pigmentation by interrupting the signalling process that follows exposure to UV radiation and ends in the creation of melanin. Vitamin C (L-ascorbic acid) is one of the best-studied ingredients in this group, which also includes vitamin E and resveratrol.

There is another group of ingredients that doesn't reduce the build-up of age spots, but 'flushes' melanin from the skin. Alpha hydroxy acid (AHA) peels, using glycolic acid and lactic acid at high concentrations, have been shown to be effective in reducing pigmentation.

Vitamin A, too, has good evidence and is commonly used; it's just harder to put into any one category, because it increases skin-cell turnover, it has some weak tyrosinase-controlling effect, and it's also an antioxidant.

As my forties recede further behind me, age spots have started to make an appearance. Creating an ESK regime to manage them has been one of our toughest tasks. While some of our best results have been with users who had previously 'tried everything' but could not budge their hyperpigmentation, there are some for whom it hasn't worked. My bet is that, both for us and the wider skincare industry, this will be one of the areas in skin that will receive a lot of research attention in the years to come.

What anti-aging procedures are available?

A lot of my patients assume I'll be injecting Botox and fillers. I don't inject them into patients, and I don't use them myself. I also don't use dermabrasion. Not laser. Not anything. I haven't even had a facial for 10 years! But they do have pretty good evidence for many skin conditions, so let's take a look at them.

Botox

This is when your face is injected with small quantities of botulinum toxin; yes, the toxin from the same *Clostridium botulinum* bacteria that gives you botulism! The toxin basically paralyses muscles, so when it's injected into specific overactive muscles around your face, it results in relaxation of those muscles. That in turn smooths the overlying skin and reduces wrinkles. Botox injections, especially when done into the upper third of the face, give you pretty predictable results, have few adverse effects and generally give high patient satisfaction.

Botulinum toxin, as Botox, was first approved by the American FDA for cosmetic use back in 2002. It was specifically licensed to treat glabellar complex muscles that form frown lines in 2013. The glabellar complex is the group of muscles at the bottom of your forehead that mainly contracts downwards, making you frown. It was also licensed to treat the lateral orbicularis oculi muscles that surround your eyes and form crow's feet wrinkles.

Botox has the most dramatic effect for people with what we call 'dynamic wrinkles' (these appear only when you laugh or frown). It also works on static wrinkles (they are always there, no matter what) but not as brilliantly; it might take a few injections and the results won't last as long — it generally needs to be redone every 12 weeks.

There are a whole lot of reasons *not* to have Botox injections. Unrealistic expectations is a big one. Botox is not going to make you look 22. Scarring, and also certain skin conditions at the injection site, such as rosacea, can make Botox a no-no for some people. Occasionally users get a droopy eye, which is not a good look, but does go away over time.

Microdermabrasion

This is basically aggressive exfoliation. The beautician or aesthetician uses a minimally abrasive instrument to gently sand your skin, removing the thicker, uneven outer layer. It might help generate more collagen in the skin. Microdermabrasion is most effective for superficial skin conditions, as it only targets the upper layers of the skin. Superficial skin conditions include fine lines and large pore size. Risks of microdermabrasion include rebound pigmentation where you actually get pigmentation spots where you've had the microdermabrasion done. It is most likely to happen if your skin tans easily and doesn't burn much.

You should avoid waxing, electrolysis and laser hair removal for one week before microdermabrasion, and either avoid sun exposure or wear a really good sunscreen for two weeks before and three weeks after the procedure. You can feel like you've been sunburned for about three days afterwards. Make sure you avoid AHAs and vitamin A skincare products for three days after microdermabrasion.

Laser skin resurfacing (also called laser peel, laser vaporisation and lasabrasion)

This is your go-to skin procedure for aging. Fractionated skin-rejuvenation lasers create microscopic heat columns that cause areas of thermal damage known as microscopic thermal zones (MTZs). The heat that is generated by the laser seems to help your skin make more collagen. The lasers specifically create MTZs with intervening normal untreated skin areas between. The areas of untouched skin act as reservoirs for tissue regeneration and remodelling. This 'fractional approach' is what allows the skin to heal much faster than if the entire area was treated, making for a quicker recovery period with less complications. Multiple sessions are needed in most cases, with about 15–25 per cent of the skin being lasered per session.

Fractional lasers can be either ablative or non-ablative. Ablative fractional lasers have longer wavelengths (in the range of 2940 to 10600nm) and lead to full thickness destruction of skin. On the other hand, non-ablative fractional lasers have wavelengths ranging from 1320 to 1927nm and don't destroy the stratum corneum. Ablative fractional lasers achieve greater efficacy in terms of anti-aging, but have a longer recovery time and higher risk of complications. These can range from rashes and infection to pigmentation and even scarring.

Laser skin resurfacing can improve the appearance of:

- Fine lines and wrinkles around and under your eyes, forehead and mouth
- Scars from acne or chickenpox
- Pigmentation spots
- General complexion
- Enlarged oil glands on the nose

When the treatment first came out it was very expensive, but the prices are coming down. I've seen some amazing results, and am thinking of getting it done myself!

Dermal fillers

Fillers are very popular, and their popularity increases year on year. You can see why: they offer the rejuvenative and 'aesthetic improvements' previously only achievable with surgery, but at a much lower cost and with little to no recovery time. They're mainly used to 'fill' deep wrinkles (called rhytides and folds), as well as to correct the soft-tissue loss that is seen as part of the aging process. These days they're used most often for cheek and chin 'augmentation', tear-trough correction, nose reshaping, 'mid-facial volumisation', lip enhancement, hand rejuvenation and the correction of facial asymmetry.

There are a few different types of fillers on the market. 'Moderate duration' biodegradable fillers, such as collagen and hyaluronic acid fillers, are reabsorbed by the body and generally last somewhere between six and

18 months, depending on the product used. These days, you can also get fillers with biodegradable particles that stimulate the body to produce its own collagen, as well as synthetic polymers that cause an inflammatory response in your skin, which, in turn, causes collagen deposition. These seem to last longer — around two years or so. And you can get non-biodegradable fillers such as polymethylmethacrylate. These are meant to be permanent, so if you do get a complication they're harder to deal with.

They do have side effects. All can cause bruising, swelling, redness and infections. The skin of patients of colour has a tendency to respond to trauma with pigmentation. Dermal fillers are a real risk for hyperpigmentation in people who tan easily and don't tend to burn. When fillers are incorrectly injected into the superficial dermis or epidermis, a bluish tinge to the skin might occur. One of my patients tried fillers and they turned into little hard balls that fell to the bottom of her face. This can definitely be a result of poor technique.

Chemical peels

In this procedure a chemical solution is applied to the skin, causing it to exfoliate and eventually peel off. The new skin cells are smoother and less wrinkled than the old skin that has been exfoliated. On the downside, the fresh skin is also temporarily more sensitive to the sun and can look a bit red and blistered, depending on the type of peel you go for.

There are three basic types of chemical peels:

- Superficial peel (the 'lunchtime peel'). AHA or another mild acid is used to exfoliate only the outer layer of skin. This is pretty effective for improving the appearance of mild skin pigmentation as well as smoothing rough skin. You heal in about a week and can wear make-up the next day.

- Medium peel. Glycolic or trichloroacetic acid (TCA) is applied to penetrate the outer and middle layers of skin to exfoliate and remove damaged skin cells. The treatment is used for age spots, fine lines and wrinkles, as well as for smoothing rough skin. This can also help treat some precancerous skin growths (actinic keratosis). The skin peels off in seven to 10 days and is healed in about 14 days.

♦ Deep peel. Trichloroacetic acid or phenol is applied to deeply penetrate the middle layer of skin to exfoliate and remove damaged skin cells. The treatment removes moderate lines, age spots, freckles and shallow scars, from acne for example. It's going to give you a dramatic improvement in skin appearance on your face, but it can only can be performed once. It takes 21 days to heal and you need to be *extremely* diligent with sunscreen for six months.

One issue with peels is that they can reactivate cold sores. So, if you're prone to cold sores, you will often be given an antiviral medication to take for one to three weeks to prevent this.

Platelet-rich plasma injections ('vampire facials')

Basically, what happens here is you get some blood taken from your arm. The blood is then put into a machine that separates it into layers, one of which has a high concentration of platelets. This 'platelet-rich plasma' is then re-injected into your skin. These facials are sold as having powers to reduce wrinkles and deep creases, plump up sagging skin, improve your complexion and reduce acne scars.

Their popularity has run way ahead of any scientific evidence to back them up.

A systematic review published in the journal *Aesthetic Plastic Surgery* by researchers in China concluded, based on studies in humans and test tubes, that platelet-rich plasma injections might play a role in promoting tissue regeneration and growing new blood vessels. It also found evidence of actual skin damage.

Another study in 2018 noted the skin inflammation as well as the formation of tiny superficial blood vessels, which can look terrible. And the authors mused: 'In the long term, the presence of inflammation and microangiopathy [AKA new blood vessels] caused by PRP injection could lead to . . . the precocious [premature] aging process.'

So I just don't think we're there yet with this one. I'd stick to the better-studied procedures.

Micro-needling

A device is used to roll tiny needles over your skin! As each fine needle punctures the skin, it creates a tiny skin wound. These controlled injuries trigger the body to heal by producing new collagen and elastin. In addition, new capillaries in the dermis are formed. These processes seem to help reduce scars, as well as contribute to improved skin texture, firmness and hydration. Like the other procedures, this is used for fine lines, wrinkles, rough skin texture and pigmentation. But it is less dramatic and causes less skin damage and downtime. It might be a better option if you have to work and can't take time off, or if you have sensitive skin or a low pain threshold. Each procedure takes anywhere from 10 minutes to an hour and can be done again around six weeks later. As after any procedure, your skin can be a bit red and sensitive for a few days and you need to be diligent with your sunscreen for several weeks.

HRT

In studies, HRT increases epidermal and dermal thickness, increases collagen and elastin content of the skin and improves skin moisture, leading to fewer wrinkles. It decreases wrinkles by stimulating the synthesis of collagen and hyaluronic acid by the fibroblasts in the dermis, and improves skin hydration and barrier function, making your skin less dry.

While, back in the 1980s, we used to put women on HRT just to look more youthful, post WHI we don't do that anymore. I know I have panned the study from here to hell and back. But looking youthful is not enough of a reason to use a medication that might have complications — albeit far fewer than were initially thought. But if you have hot flushes and you need to take HRT for them, you'll delay and even reverse skin aging.

If you don't need HRT, don't worry: scientists have your back! Work is being done investigating topical oestrogen and creams, as well as skin-specific selective oestrogen receptor modulators. These might one day hold the key to optimal skin health and youthful looks in the post-menopausal period.

Are there lifestyle changes I can make to combat aging?

There are stacks of evidence building for how your diet influences the appearance of aging in your face. Findings from a few, albeit pretty small, studies suggest that a diet packed with plenty of fresh fruits and vegetables might help prevent damage that leads to premature skin aging.

Specifically, a diet high in vitamin C and linoleic acid (the main poly-unsaturated fat found in vegetable oil, nuts and seeds) is linked to more youthful skin. And, on the flip side, a diet containing lots of sugar or other refined carbohydrates and dietary fat can accelerate aging.

One US study found that women with a wrinkled appearance had diets lower in vitamin A and protein. Vitamin A is found in a pretty diverse range of foods, from broccoli and spinach to yellow veggies and dairy. The richest source is liver. The American Academy of Dermatology recommends taking your diet in a healthier direction as a pretty good idea for aging skin.

On the negative side, I'm amazed at how few studies have directly looked at links between drinking alcohol and aging skin. It is believed that alcohol causes a stress reaction in the skin that can contribute to skin aging. Anecdotally, drinkers often look a lot older and, stopping the drink, or just easing up, seems to have a great impact on the skin. Warning: this is my opinion; it's not scientifically validated!

Get enough sleep: this is not only a good idea in theory, but proven. Studies indicate that chronic poor sleep quality (we're talking less than 5 hours of decent sleep a night) is associated with increased visible signs of aging, diminished skin-barrier function and lower satisfaction with appearance.

Can I get beauty from supplements?

It stands to reason that if the intake of key nutrients has a powerful effect on the appearance of the face, maybe supplements can help. We're just not there yet. One study compared the facial features of women taking various supplements with those who took none. Supplement use was not signifi-cantly associated with the reduction of any visible signs of skin aging, the researchers found.

And yet, the market is growing exponentially. When we go to the enormous Cosmoprof conference in Hong Kong each year, the number of 'nutraceutical' stalls, and the interest from buyers, increases dramatically year on year. What is a nutraceutical? It's a new-age term that captures nutritional supplements based on a food that give — or claim to give — some sort of medical effect. It can be for depression, memory or beauty. They're largely unregulated. So far, the human trials that have been done (and there are lots) are interesting, but you couldn't call them conclusive. In some cases, the ingredient tested is part of a complex cocktail, so who knows what the active ingredient actually is? In other cases, clinical trials were too small to have any statistical power and many didn't have a placebo group for comparison. With that in mind, below are the studies we *do* have.

Collagen supplements

There are lots of these on the market, so getting your head around them can be a tall order. Luckily for us, dermatologists from the University of California Irvine did a review of the published studies of collagen supplements for wound healing and skin aging in 2019. The authors examined 11 studies, with a total of 805 patients, that had lasted between four and 12 weeks. The results from those trials were pretty exciting for both short- and long-term use of oral collagen supplements for wound healing and skin aging. They appear to increase skin elasticity, hydration and the amount of collagen in the skin. They were also safe, with no reports of side effects.

Peptides

Peptides are short protein chains formed by a few amino acids and with a low molecular weight. Those used for cosmetic purposes are typically derived from collagen. These 'nutraceuticals' make pretty huge claims about their anti-aging properties. Quite a few small trials have been done. All were sponsored by whatever company made the peptide combo being studied, so that makes the studies a little dodgy. But all had some pretty impressive results. After around 12 weeks, researchers were seeing better skin elasticity and more collagen.

Vitamins

Four studies have found a link between short-term supplementation of high doses of vitamin C in combination with vitamin E, which showed a positive correlation with more youthful-looking skin.

In a separate trial, a cocktail of vitamins C and E, along with a blend of other supplements, was studied in 60 people for 90 days. Results showed a significant improvement in skin elasticity, moisture and antioxidant capacity. There was no placebo arm, so it's hard to know what to make of this tiny study.

Polyunsaturated fatty acids (PUFAs)

Traditionally used to treat eczema and psoriasis, a couple of studies of fish oils have been done for protection against UV radiation. The results have been OK, but the studies are too small to be really convincing.

Polysaccharides

Polysaccharides are complex sugar molecules with both structural and energy-storage functions. In one study of polysaccharides combined with vitamin C and zinc, people taking the combo had less wrinkles, mottled skin, dryness and brittleness of hair and nails, as well as more skin elasticity and thickness after 90 days. Other commercial preparations of polysaccharides, often from fish or marine-cartilage origin, have similar positive results. But again, we're talking small trials and the manufacturer sponsored the trials.

Carotenoids

These nutrients are well-known antioxidants and include alpha-, gamma- and beta-carotene, lutein, zeaxanthin and lycopene. They have been well studied for their effects on everything from age-related macular degeneration to cardiovascular disease. Several studies have shown nicely that supplements of carotenoids can prevent UV-induced skin damage.

I find these supplements interesting. They're not commercial products so you can say the trials of carotenoids are independent. And they did show protection from sun damage, including burning. The supplements are not great quality though and many people taking them reported that their skin turned yellow!

What skincare ingredients should I *not* waste my money on?

In most cases we don't have evidence to say conclusively that something *doesn't* work. We often have no evidence at all. But these ones have been *proven* to be a total waste of money — assume these both get a three-Gwyneth score.

Coenzyme Q10 (ubiquinone)

There's been lots of interest in this antioxidant. Especially because one form of it seems to prevent breakdown of fats. The problem is the molecule size is so big you can't get it into the skin if applied in a skincare product. Studied extensively and found to be ineffective against skin aging.

Hyaluronic acid in skin care

While it is an essential ingredient *inside* the skin for hydration and texture, putting hyaluronic acid *on* the face, in any form, is a waste of time. Studies show it can't penetrate the epidermis and breaks down rapidly.

Why am I getting acne and breakouts at menopause?

I've already mentioned that I've never had a time of life without breakouts. From the day I turned 11 to today, pimples have been constant companions. Under 30 it was just straight acne; I have now been diagnosed with rosacea. And, given how common rosacea is, and how few of my patients know they have it, I thought it would be worth dealing with pimples that happen later in life.

Adult female acne has been traditionally defined as acne in women over 25 years of age. Adult acne is on the rise, affecting up to 15 per cent of women.

But there's also a pretty good chance that your 'acne' could be rosacea. Dr Eleni Yiasemides is a consultant dermatologist in Sydney. Because I send so many patients to her, I sought her advice when writing this book. She told me that she has a lot of patients referred with 'new acne' (or acne that has 'come back' at perimenopause after 20–30 years). 'It's nearly always rosacea,' she said. While estimates vary, it's thought that 10 per cent of the population have rosacea. It is most common in fair-skinned women aged 30–50, but especially around the time of menopause.

Whether you have acne or rosacea, it's no fun. And, if you're like me, getting the breakouts under control will make you feel a whole lot better (and probably shrink your make-up bill).

Have I got acne, or rosacea?

Hands down, the best way to know which you have is to visit a dermatologist. If you can't wait to see a specialist and want to have a better understanding of what's happening with your skin, here are some of the things to look for.

	ACNE	ROSACEA
Pimple/pustule appearance	Blackheads, whiteheads, pimples or painful cysts	Pimple-like, but with no blackheads, which is a critical difference
Pimple/pustule location	Face, especially chin and jawline (also neck, upper back, chest and shoulders)	Face (also scalp, neck, chest and upper back). Rosacea tends to always come back in the same place
Oiliness	T zone of the face (T shape across forehead, down nose and chin)	Often 'combination skin'. Often not especially oily
Redness	Around each pimple only	Often on cheeks, forehead, nose or chin. Can be occasional or permanent redness, depending on the type of rosacea
Blood vessels	Nothing unusual	Sometimes visible on some part of the face
Skin sensitivity	Not especially	Usually sensitive skin. Particularly to some make-up and skincare products
Who is likely to get it?	Generally teens and twenties (found in older people up to 50, but never beyond 50)	Generally fair-skinned people over 30 (and especially around menopause)

You're probably looking at the table and thinking, I am not sure that I can tell the difference — and you would be in good company. That's why it is so commonly mis/under-diagnosed. To make things more complicated, there are four distinctly different types of rosacea. You would usually only have one, but they can progress from one to the other. Occasionally, you can be unlucky and have different types at the same time.

- Type 1: Flushing (erythematotelangiectatic) rosacea. Flushing and persistent redness, particularly in the middle of the face (may also include visible blood vessels). Skin is often sensitive.

- Type 2: Pustular (papulopustular) rosacea. Persistent redness with bumps and pimples that flare up. Skin is often sensitive.

- Type 3: Thickened skin (phymatous) rosacea. Thickened and uneven skin on the nose and also chin, ears, eyelids and forehead. Think of the big red nose on men, which is traditionally associated with drinking but is actually just a form of rosacea.

- Type 4: Eye (ocular) rosacea. Eye irritations including dry eye, tearing, redness, burning, swollen, crusty eyelids, styes and sometimes vision loss.

How should I treat my rosacea?

How you manage it will depend on the type of rosacea. A good dermatologist is the place to start. They can prescribe a number of different medications or light therapies.

That said, if you have types 1 or 2 rosacea (the most common forms), there are four things you can do yourself:

Avoid triggers

There are a number of things that commonly trigger a flare-up and increase sensitivity. It's best to try to avoid these:

- Very hot or cold temperatures, rapid changes in temperature, and dry air are all common triggers — best to try to avoid them.

- Stress and anxiety can cause flare-ups; so, as well as being good for your overall wellbeing to avoid these, it will help manage your rosacea symptoms.

- Your own special triggers can vary, from particular foods (especially spicy ones) to strenuous exercise. Caffeine and alcohol are often blamed, but the evidence for these as triggers is mixed.

- Avoid microdermabrasion, chemical peels and certain ingredients in skin care such as alcohol, exfoliators (physical or chemical, such as AHAs), menthol and some essential oils that can lead to flare-ups.

- UV and sun exposure are the most common aggravating factors for rosacea, so wearing a hat, staying out of the sun and wearing sunscreen daily are recommended. Zinc-based sunscreens are recommended because they deflect heat away from the skin and are less irritating generally.

Stop smoking

Smokers get more acne, and smokers with acne are always advised to quit. Weirdly, they don't get more rosacea. But just stop anyway because it's so bad for you!

Fix your diet

There is some evidence that consuming cow's milk (interestingly, especially skim milk!) and having a diet high in sugar is linked to a higher rate of acne. For rosacea, the story is more complex. Apart from your triggers, rosacea seems to have a pretty high correlation with gut disorders. Research from Denmark has linked rosacea to conditions as diverse as inflammatory bowel disease, such as Crohn's disease, and *Helicobacter pylorii*, the bug that causes stomach ulcers. In one small study of 40 people, researchers found that patients with rosacea were 13 times more likely to have small intestinal bacterial overgrowth (SIBO). They reported that treating SIBO with antibiotics led to remission of rosacea in 100 per cent of cases. Even more amazingly, they followed up the people for three years and still none had rosacea. Now SIBO can be fixed not just with antibiotics. Adding fibre to the diet can help.

Eczema has been treated in trials with combinations of prebiotics and probiotics. The race is now on to see if we get the same benefits for people with rosacea.

Regardless, a healthy diet is currently advocated as a way of having a healthy gut microbiome and a reduction in inflammatory conditions, possibly including rosacea.

Choose your skincare products carefully

Rosacea leads to inflamed, irritated and sensitive skin. So, management should include products and ingredients that don't irritate, but help improve the barrier function of the skin. And, where relevant, using a gentle ingredient that can help with the pimples is great. Happily, there are some ingredients that should fit the bill.

Because so many people with rosacea have super-sensitive skin, it's a good idea to patch-test any skincare products first. Do this by applying it behind the ear and on the side of the neck. Most dermatologists recommend you avoid products with any significant amount of alcohol (if it appears as one of the first few ingredients listed), witch hazel, fragrances, menthol, peppermint and eucalyptus oils. Dr Yiasemides also suggests avoiding masks and scrubs — they can be very irritating. If you can, choose skincare products with a slightly acidic pH (below 7). The skin's pH is somewhere between 4.1 and 5.8 (average 4.7), so it's acidic. Using alkaline products leads to moisture loss, irritation and pressure on the skin to bring the pH back down to its normal level. Most manufacturers won't reveal the pH of their products, so you may have to ask — somewhere in the 4–6 range is ideal.

- Gentle cleanser. If you like that 'squeaky' clean feeling after a cleanse, that's because your cleanser removes lots of grease and fats. With your sensitive skin, that's the first thing that should change. If you can find a gentle soap-free cleanser that you like, that's a great start.
- Vitamin B3. Niacinamide improves and repairs the barrier function of the skin and has anti-inflammatory properties. So it helps calm skin and improve its ability to retain moisture. It has also been shown to specifically assist in managing rosacea symptoms.

- Vitamin A or retinoids. Retinoids are effective and are often used in the treatment of types 1 and 2 rosacea. However, prescription forms of vitamin A that have the strongest evidence can be irritating, especially on sensitive rosacea skin. Dr Yiasemides suggests starting gently and building up the dose slowly. The most effective and least irritating alternative is the non-prescription form of vitamin A, retinal. (We include retinal in our ESK Ultimate A and Ultimate A+ night creams.)

- Moisturise. Skin that has a compromised barrier function can get dry and sensitive. So, keeping your skin moisturised will help.

Why am I growing chin hair?

Grrrr! I hate chin hairs. As the hair on our heads starts thinning, the hair on our face starts sprouting, and continues to get worse with age. Well, it does for 50 per cent of us, which is the number of women who reach menopause with facial hair we didn't have before.

When it comes to your face, androgens can transform hair follicles from the soft fuzzy 'vellus' variety, to thicker, coarser and darker 'terminal' follicles. Thus the hair is transformed into coarser and wirier hair — much like pubic hair. These 'terminal hairs' (which are *double* the thickness of the softer, fluffier 'vellus' hairs) make your chin hairs, and the occasional hair on your top lip, look and feel awful. Oestrogen makes facial hair softer and smoother. The determination of what hormone receptors grow on which hair follicles, on which body part, and in what number, is determined largely by your genes. So, the hormones coursing through your body might be normal in their levels, but if there are more receptors on follicles to be activated, you can get facial hair growing anyway!

We learned in Chapter 2 that oestrogen increases the liver's production of sex hormone-binding globulin (SHBG). And this, in turn, 'binds' up androgens such as testosterone, and keeps them from being too active. As oestrogen falls, so too does SHBG, and androgens just float around in the bloodstream unbound and available to start activating testosterone receptors everywhere. The increase in active androgens circulating in the body is no longer counteracted by oestrogens. More free-riding testosterone means more chin hairs, and hair loss from your head! Another thing that impacts on SHBG is insulin — the higher your insulin level, the lower your SHBG — so being overweight can cause more chin hairs to sprout as well. If your menopause has come packaged up with weight gain around your middle, that's a double risk for chin hair. And, once primed, testosterone receptors on hair-producing cells can continue to be active long after testosterone levels fall.

How can I get rid of my facial hair?

Shaving, bleaching and chemical depilators are very effective to *temporarily* nix those unwanted hairs. Shaving can lead to a blunt hair end, but, although that can feel like stubble, it does not *encourage* extra hair growth as we are often told.

Don't knock bleaching either. If you only have a few hairs, localised to one area, it might be all you need. Depilating agents aren't always as effective. For a start, they can give many women a nasty skin irritation, and studies have found they actually make rebound hair growth worse! Doctors warn you against plucking and/or waxing because of the risk of a little folliculitis infection. Plus trauma to the hair shaft can cause the subsequent development of ingrown hairs and skin damage.

Zap them

There are marvellous methods of permanent hair removal these days. Laser hair removal is best on dark hair, so if you have grey chin or face hairs it mightn't be as successful. This is because the success of the treatment requires the energy from the laser to be absorbed by the pigments in the hairs and converted to heat, which damages the follicle. No pigment in the hair, less damage to the follicles. If you have grey hair, you might be better off with electrolysis, which damages the terminal hair follicles. The problem is finding someone who can do it for you — beauticians experienced in electrolysis seem to be few and far between.

Eflornithine

This is a cream you rub on hairy parts of your face twice a day; it slows down hair growth but it's not cheap and, as soon as you stop using it, the hairs start growing back. It starts working in around six weeks and gets to full effect at about six months. You can use it combined with laser or electrolysis if you want.

Medications

Available on prescription, medications for excess facial hair (and thinning hair on your head) are pretty effective. They include androgen receptor blockers, such as the diuretic spironolactone, and cyproterone acetate. All drugs that block androgen action will give you similar results.

I've got hair on my chin, but the hair on my head is thinning! Help!

Less than 45 per cent of women will go through life with a full head of hair. Luckily, only 1 per cent of us suffer severe hair loss. But none of us likes losing our luscious locks. There are two known factors involved in thinning hair: androgen levels and genetic predisposition. Androgens can also transform large terminal hair follicles into small vellus hair follicles on the scalp, especially in genetically predisposed women. Can you believe the irony of hair follicles swapping roles, putting vellus hair on your head and terminal hair on your face? We still have no idea why this happens! But there is more to it than simply androgens. Blood levels of androgens have little to do with hair loss.

You should start treatment for this sooner rather than later: by the time you have noticed the hair loss, it is already pretty advanced. Treatment usually takes one to two years to start working. And, once you have started, treatments need to continue indefinitely to maintain the effect.

HRT

Female-pattern hair loss worsens after menopause, but sadly there's no proven help from HRT. So, if you're taking HRT, you should sleep better, flush less, have healthier bones and a more youthful vagina and face, but the hair on your head won't care!

Minoxidil

The most commonly used non-hormonal treatment for androgenetic alopecia in men and women is Minoxidil, a lotion you rub onto your scalp every day. It was initially a drug for hypertension, but lost popularity because a major side effect was hypertrichosis — excessive hair growth! It then had a marketing makeover and was reinvented as an anti-hair-loss product. To this day we still don't really understand how it works.

Dr Eleni Yiasemides told me that Minoxidil won't completely fix the problem, but it will limit how bad it gets. She warns that you need to persist because it takes a few months to see any effects.

Hair transplant

I hope you've saved up. This is a time-consuming and very expensive undertaking. The idea is to take hairs from the base and sides of your scalp and transplant them to the top, where the hair is thinning. It works, but it's unaffordable for lots of women.

Is it an illusion, or is my nose getting bigger as I age?

My grandma was an absolute beauty in her twenties, thirties and forties. Slim, with a beautiful face; I could look at photos of her in her wedding dress all day. But by the time I met her, she was in her sixties and I remember her having a really big nose. It sure was not there in those wedding pictures. So, did grandma's nose just grow and grow? Despite incorrect information you might have seen or read, the nose actually *stops* growing during your teen years. But it certainly does change shape and this happens for a few reasons.

Firstly, the cartilage part of the nose becomes weaker, making the tip of your nose droop so it looks longer or a bit 'hooked'. This is called tip ptosis.

The skin of your nose actually becomes thinner, but the sebaceous glands that produce the oil and sebum become more prominent. This changes the nature of the skin so that it looks both heavier and full of tiny veins. And it contributes further to that nasal tip droop. The facial bones that support the nose, the maxilla bones, along with the tissues that overlie them, your cheeks and lips, are slowly reabsorbed and they actually start to shrink. This makes the nose, which doesn't shrink, look more prominent.

You don't need to do anything about this. Your nose will still work (although smell does diminish with age, regardless of what your nose looks like) so try to just embrace your new nose.

If you'd like another option, there are plenty out there. You'd need to go to a plastic surgeon if you wanted to discuss surgical options for nose remodelling (rhinoplasty).

Why have my boobs got so saggy?

Dr Amira Sanki is a plastic surgeon and a member of the Australasian Society of Aesthetic Plastic Surgeons. I have referred patients to her for years, including patients on *Embarrassing Bodies Down Under*, and she has a special interest in women's bodies around menopause. She sees many women who hit menopause, gain a lot of weight and get much bustier as a result. And bigger boobs sag more. Which is pretty ironic. 'Younger women just want bigger boobs,' she told me. 'Older women often just want convenience.' And enormous boobs are often incredibly inconvenient. It's not just about sagging — you can usually get a bra to hide that pretty easily under your clothes — but large breasts give you headaches; back, neck and shoulder pain; and require you to wear enormous, unsexy bras.

Breast tissue consists of glandular tissue that makes milk for an infant and fatty tissue. As you go through menopause, your breasts change and you get a lot more fatty breast tissue and less glandular tissue. As the breasts lose exposure to oestrogen, the connective tissues that support the breasts become less elastic and the fatty breast tissue doesn't have any support. Hello, saggy boobs! Studies using MRI machines prove two fairly consistent changes after menopause. Firstly, your nipples start pointing south; surgically, we call it 'caudal nipple deviation', although I'm not sure that sounds any better. Secondly, after menopause your boobs get bigger, even if you don't gain weight.

Breast surgery

If you do decide to have surgery to change your breasts, that is your business and nobody else's. Dr Sanki told me most patients she sees undergo this surgery for themselves and themselves alone. It is basically never about pleasing a partner, even a new partner. I wish more studies were done on this, because anecdotally this is pretty different to younger women who are trying to conform to a perceived beauty ideal.

Breast-reduction surgery (often with nipple relocation or mastopexy and breast lift) is the cosmetic surgery procedure with the highest degree of patient satisfaction. So, if anyone wants to give you a hard time about it, just ignore them.

What's happened to my labia?

Yes, I am going there. Yes, the labia majora (the 'outer lips') sag after menopause. They actually don't get any bigger with age; they stay more or less the same size from puberty to old age. Which is significant, because after menopause all the other genital tissues, from inner lips to clitoris, start to shrink. The labia majora just get saggier.

Dr Jennifer Gunter is a Canadian gynaecologist and blogger. 'The lower genital tract is built to stretch (a good thing for having babies),' she says. 'But gravity takes its toll on stretchy tissues. So, your labia might possibly wrinkle a little more than everything else because they are a bit more elastic.' Dr Sanki points out that after menopause most women lose their labial fat. 'So the labia majora can feel like empty bags of skin,' she says. Women who have permanently removed their pubic hair will have labia that appear more prominent as well, Dr Gunter adds.

Fixing saggy labia

I don't want to be too judgey here; being judgemental of my sisters is the last thing I want to be. But, seriously? In my own very personal experience as a GP, the women who want their labia 'fixed' have been through a trauma. Maybe their partner had an affair — well, that would be the most common — and they want sexier labia to re-engage their partner. Studies tell us that women seeking labiaplasty (surgery to reduce the size of labia) have often received a negative comment about their labia from a partner. I haven't met a woman who undertakes this surgery just for her own enjoyment. Unlike your boobs, you don't look at your own labia often. Ladies, if your partner has cheated on you because your labia weren't 'pretty' enough, does he really deserve you?

So I mention labiaplasty here, but under duress. Because I think you should love your labia, with their crinkles and sagging and grey pubic hair. And anyone privileged enough to see them, because *you let them,* should shut the hell up.

Labiaplasty is plastic surgery to trim the labia, and can be done to the labia majora or minora. You *can* do this; I really don't think you *should.* Larger labia don't give you thrush or limit sexual satisfaction. I think advertising this procedure should be banned. I consider it genital mutilation. I think unless you're a professional cyclist who is finding the size of her labia career-limiting, the entire procedure should be shunned out of existence. And now I'll stop ranting.

Why have I suddenly got tuckshop-lady arms?

Loss of subcutaneous fat (under the skin) causes sagginess, and that includes the skin under your arms. In terms of the role hormones play versus simply aging, it's hard to be 100 per cent certain, as doing a study to control for both is hard. But we don't tend to hear about tuckshop-men arms. So I'm backing the menopause a bit here. And probably your genes — although that's never been studied. 'Even skinny women get saggy arm skin,' says Dr Sanki. Sure, if your skin has been stretched by your being overweight, it will be worse. But it's not the only issue. 'The dermis on the undersides of the arms is very thin,' Dr Sanki told me. 'In fact, it's 30 per cent less thick and strong than the skin of your breasts!'

That makes fixing saggy arms a surgical challenge. That thin, crepey skin rules out liposuction as the skin is too thin to cope with it. Instead, if you want to get rid of saggy arm skin, you'll need surgery. A brachioplasty is not for the faint-hearted: we're talking about surgically removing the excess fat and skin from armpit to elbow.

'One thing that's great about surgery when you're older is that you get a much better scar,' Dr Sanki told me. This is a function of a slightly less enthusiastic immune system, leading to a smaller build-up of keloid scar tissue.

And — I've got a double chin and jowls!

That subcutaneous fat loss that comes from age and hormones can affect the area under your chin, too. Although men get jowly as much as women so age is probably a bigger factor than menopause per se! Gravity is not your friend when it comes to saggy skin on your chin. A couple of other things contribute as well: the superior and inferior jowl fat pads start to shrink with age and literally slide downwards. Plus, the skin under the chin is really thin naturally, so can't resist the extra weight of the fat pads that have slid downwards.

If this bothers you, fat-busting injections of deoxycholic acid can be given into the 'submental' region under the chin to dissolve the fat. Deoxycholic acid is actually a bile acid that plays a role in digestion by emulsifying fats. This treatment can be a bit gruelling. A single treatment is up to 50 injections, and up to six treatments are needed, each one at least one month apart. As far as fat dissolving goes, it works pretty well. Mind you, that won't help with saggy skin, which can look even worse afterwards. This is probably better for younger people with thicker, bouncier skin.

Dermal fillers can also do wonders for rejuvenating the jaw line. Or you could have surgical correction as a part of a 'face lift'. In one technique, entering your skin from inside the mouth, the fallen cheek fat pads are located and then removed!

Why have I got droopy eyelids and eye bags?

Dermatochalasis is an excess of lax, stretched eyelid skin and muscle (both upper and lower lids), which gives your eyes a 'baggy' appearance. The eyelid is actually one of the first areas of the face to show the effects of aging in both men and women. This is caused by a combination of gravity and loss of skin elasticity, along with weakening of the eyelid connective tissues, and it is more than just a cosmetic issue. Dermatochalasis also often obstructs your vision. At night as your pupil dilates, the saggy upper lid can simply get in the way. Plus, it can cause entropion of the upper eyelid (the eyelid folds inwards and the eyelashes irritate the eyeball) and ectropion of the lower eyelid (the sagging outwards of the lid leaves the delicate inner eyelid skin exposed and easily irritated).

It often comes packaged up with steatoblepharon. This is a forward herniation of the under-eye fat pad, giving you really major bags under the eyes. The most effective treatment is surgical, and you can get some really wonderful results.

Why are my nails suddenly brittle?

I turned, once again, to consultant dermatologist Dr Eleni Yiasemides. We know menopause causes brittle nails, and yet it hasn't been studied formally. 'Your nails are just an extension of your skin,' she explained. So, they are prone to drying out and brittleness, and are therefore easily damaged. She has this advice for better looking nails:

- Keep them short. Short nails are less likely to snag on things and tear.
- Avoid protracted contact with harsh cleaning products that can further dry out the nails.
- Use petroleum jelly on your cuticles. Eleni points out that care of your cuticles will be critical for the development of a healthy nail.

MAKE ME LOOK LIKE HELEN MIRREN

THE BOTTOM LINE

This is not of interest to every woman. But my passion is your empowerment to choose. And good choices need good information inputs. So here you can get armed with the information you need to look your best.

Skin is the body's protection. Everyone's skin changes as we age — muscles shrink and loosen, and subcutaneous fat disappears.

It is difficult to tell which changes are due to age and which are menopause, but studies show a woman's skin loses 30 per cent of its collagen within five years of menopause.

Sun exposure is the biggest source of aging that you can prevent, through the use of sunscreens and other lifestyle measures.

When choosing skin care such as cleansers, moisturisers, exfoliators and sunscreen, choose evidence-based products.

A diet high in vitamin C and linoleic acid (found in vegetable oil, nuts and seeds) is linked to more youthful skin. A diet containing lots of sugar, refined carbohydrates and dietary fat can accelerate aging.

Vitamin A is the most effective skincare ingredient for anti-aging (it also has evidence for management of acne and rosacea).

When vitamin C is applied to the skin, it acts as an antioxidant — it reduces and reverses pigmentation, wrinkles, fine lines and skin roughness, and protects from UV radiation. It also promotes collagen growth.

Vitamin B3, or niacinamide, is used for anti-aging, managing acne and rosacea, and reducing the risk of non-melanoma skin cancer.

EPILOGUE

The whole experience of being a woman has changed over the past 100 years. Our emancipation has brought so much, including options for managing menopause and our journey towards it.

Menopause is natural, sure. But so are tuberculosis and cockroach infestations. Feeling hot, tired, cranky, teary, itchy, unsexy, achy and bloated can all be part of the natural experience of menopause — and today you don't need to surrender to that without at least trying to make your life more bearable.

Hot flushes, experienced by 75 per cent of women around menopause, can range from mildly annoying to debilitating. For one in 20 of us they can last the rest of our lifetime. But, for most, time is a healer and the flushes will fade (the average duration is 7.4 years, although you might be lucky and only get them for a year). Vaginal symptoms — dryness, itch and discomfort, and urine leakage — will never get better and, in fact, will only get worse. Studies suggest that 80 per cent of women 65 and over have at least some vaginal menopause symptoms.

Enduring this as 'just part of getting older', women don't talk to each other about it, we sure as hell don't talk to our doctors about it, and we stop talking to our partners about it. We just wear incontinence pads and avoid sex. We give up an entire part of life as a lost cause!

We put up with insomnia (with and without the hot flushes), mood swings, aches and pains, bloating and itchy skin as well, often not connecting the dots to our hormonal stage of life, or just believing there's nothing that can be done.

As a woman, as a doctor and as someone in my fifties, I felt this book had to be written to give women power over our bodies.

You see, luckily for us, we have an enormous variety of great options for managing hot flushes. By now, I hope you are ready to at least consider hormone replacement therapy (HRT). After all, for hot flushes it is up to 98 per cent effective! That kind of efficacy is close to unheard of in medicine. If we had medication with those statistics for heart disease and diabetes, we'd all live to be 150!

So, why is HRT not embraced by everyone? When the Women's Health Initiative study first reported a link between taking HRT and developing breast cancer and heart disease in 2002, women and their doctors panicked. Suddenly a mere hot flush seemed like a trivial complaint in comparison to dying of cancer. Most women refused to take it, their doctors wouldn't prescribe it, and governments and drug companies stopped putting funds behind it. Those women who went to a doctor begging for some relief from their menopause symptoms were given an ear-bashing and, if they *did* start taking HRT, then kept their prescriptions secret. And into this abyss of mismanagement crept the opportunists. There has been an enormous rise in so called 'bio-identical hormone' treatments that falsely promise to be safer than HRT and escape scrutiny and oversight by government regulators. Then there are the peddlers of teas, vitamins and diets that simply cannot deliver on their promises and prey on the needs of vulnerable women.

What we know now, of course, is that the risks posed by taking HRT are, in fact, pretty minor. And those risks are probably only for particular women on particular forms of HRT that are rarely prescribed today. It now seems your HRT is less likely to cause breast cancer than drinking a couple of glasses of wine a night or being overweight. We now know that too many women stopped or declined HRT, preferring to put up with their symptoms than get treatment. The cost in extra bone fractures alone (oestrogen, both natural and from HRT, strengthens bones) has been massive since the study was released.

Not everyone needs HRT. If you have healthy bones, have only a couple of hot flushes a week, aren't moody or exhausted, and your vagina is pinging on overdrive, why would you bother taking a medication? If flushing is your only menopause problem and you have a strong aversion to HRT, you have other options, from simple interventions such as hypnosis, to complementary therapies and prescription drugs from your doctor. There are also multiple options to help your aging skin, your bones, your bloating, your aches and pains and even your moods.

My passion is to give you choices, empowerment and agency at this time in your life, to free you from unnecessary fear, guilt and shame, and help you enjoy this second era of your life with as much gusto as the first.

READ THIS, DEAR PARTNER

Menopause specialist Dr Fiona Jane suggested I give you a couple of pages to hand to your partner. What a brilliant idea. Let's do this Q&A style.

What is happening to my partner?

Her hormones have already changed or are currently changing. If she is in perimenopause, her hormones will be all over the shop. Perimenopause is the phase between motherly fertility and supreme matriarchal wisdom; it usually starts between the ages of 42 and 51 and lasts between two and eight years. For 30 years your beloved has had a fairly predictable hormonal cycle, but in perimenopause, her cycle frequency is changing, her oestrogen peaks and troughs are swinging wildly, and her traditional chill-out hormone, progesterone, has gone missing in action.

Medically she is quite likely to have an awesome combo of at least some of the following: insomnia, anxiety, depression, aches and pains, gut issues, irregular and perhaps heavy periods, incontinence, sore breasts, hot flushes and a dry vagina.

Some compassion would be excellent: this won't last forever, but it will probably be a few years. After menopause (marked by the one-year anniversary of her last period), most of those symptoms will go, but the hot flushes could continue, possibly get worse, and come packaged with night sweats. And her vagina and bladder might really start to give her grief. Support her in putting herself first for a while and getting some help if she needs it. There are treatments for everything, but she needs to feel valued enough to seek them out.

How long will this last?

I don't know, but I can give you stats. In most cases, time is a healer and if she waits out the symptoms they will almost always go away. The problem is, that is often a long wait. On average, hot flushes last for 7.4 years. For one in eight women, the hot flushes never end. Without treatment, her vaginal dryness and bladder problems could last forever and continue to get worse.

We're hardly ever having sex. What's going on?

There are two things that could be happening. She might have low blood testosterone levels, reducing her libido so that she's not interested in sex. And her lower oestrogen levels cause the cells of her vagina to dry out, making sex uncomfortable and even painful — so her low libido doubles down because she fears the pain associated with sex.

Neither of these things are about you. But, if left unmanaged, this is not a menopause issue that will fix itself; in fact, it's likely to get worse over time. There are medical treatments for both causes of low libido. Talk to her about what she is experiencing and try to be understanding; you can work through this together. But recognise that a lot of things are changing and perimenopause is no walk in the park. Be supportive of her getting help; not for you, but for her and for the two of you as a couple. Meanwhile, most men I know are high achievers when it comes to masturbating; so, perfect the art! Apart from anything else, it can temporarily take the tension out of a subject that can deeply affect your relationship if handled without sensitivity.

She's yelling at me all the time. What have I done?

It's not you; it's her. This is a pretty emotional time for her; it's a huge change and she's coming to terms with it. She might be sleep deprived — she's not helped by her wildly raging hormones, but that won't last forever. If your testosterone levels were swinging wildly, you'd also be moody and erratic. Try to be gentle, supporting and loving. Perhaps give the laundry and kitchen a bit more helpful attention; maybe now is a good time to take up golf and get out of the house for a while!

She's put on weight, but she won't take my advice.

Is that meant to sound ironic? I ask because, statistically speaking, more men than women are overweight. So, if you're a pot calling a kettle black, let's try changing the conversation. How about: 'We've let ourselves go a bit. Let's stop eating ice cream after dinner and go for a walk instead.' While we're at it, why don't you go to the doctor together? Midlife is a good time to get your blood pressure and cholesterol checked, and make sure you're up to date with screening such as a bowel cancer test or, in her case, a mammogram. Men are notorious doctor avoiders, so addressing this as a couple might be better.

She's a pain in the neck at night. Blankets on, blankets off, fan on and off: she's driving me crazy.

Yeah, that is totally annoying for you. But it's worse for her, I promise.

Here are your choices: you can put up with it. If you have a spare room, you can move in there. Or, in my opinion, nirvana . . . encourage her to get treatment. The night-time dance might go on for years, but we have treatments that are up to 98 per cent effective.

PS: Do you snore? You might be annoying her, too. If she's getting up frequently in the night, getting back to sleep is much harder if you are snoring. Plus, you might be at risk of serious consequences from sleep apnoea. So why not both go to the doctor and get help together? You might get to sleep in the same bed *and* have sex, too!

THANK YOU

Writing this book has been a privilege. I have so many people to thank.

Firstly, my children: you make everything worthwhile. Secondly, my husband, Daniel. I wrote this book on weekends and at night (and on a week-long writers' retreat) while working full time. That meant he got to know the local supermarket and the inside of our laundry pretty well. Daniel, you are always there with a freshly made coffee, some words of wisdom and that enormous and generous smile! And you're a crack editor.

To the many experts I leaned on for advice and guidance. In no particular order: Professor Rod Baber, Dr Nicholas Panay, Dr Tim Hillard, Dr Terri Foran, Professor Bronwyn Stuckey, Professor Martha Hickey, Professor John Eden, Dr Dean Conrad, Dr David Rosen, Dr Fiona Jane, Professor Gayle Fischer, Dr Saxon Smith, Jo Lamble, Dr Amira Sanki, Dr Eleni Yiasemides, Ginette Lenham, Michael Buckley, Giselle Sabbah and Kathryn Eastlake.

Thanks, too, to my wonderful publisher, Corinne Roberts. Corinne: this was your idea and, through your support and nurturing, we have a book that I hope will help many women. Together with Julie and Jane, the most capable and positive editors ever, making menopause a better experience for women became a passion we all shared. Thanks also to Viv, Dannielle, Kane and Garry. Working with all of you guys is a dream. Can we do another one?

Mostly, thank you to every one of my menopausal patients. You have shared your stories, and been generous and honest. You are brave, fierce, at times vulnerable, and always inspiring. I feel so lucky to share your journeys and learn from you.

FURTHER READING
AND REFERENCES

I consulted hundreds of scientific studies, articles, websites and books for *The M Word*. If you'd like to read further, the online articles and organisations listed below are a great place to start. For a complete list of references, please visit the Murdoch Books website (murdochbooks.com.au) and search for *The M Word*.

Articles

Davis, S.R., MBBS, PhD, Baber, R., B.Pharm, MBBS, FRANZCOG, et al, 'Global consensus position statement on the use of testosterone therapy for women', *Climacteric*, 2019

de Villiers, T.J., Hall, J.E., et al, 'Revised global consensus statement on menopausal hormone therapy', *Climacteric*, 20 June 2016

Jin, J., MD, MPH, 'Vaginal and urinary symptoms of menopause', *JAMA: The Journal of the American Medical Association*, 4 April 2017

Lobo, R.A., 'Where are we 10 years after the Women's Health Initiative?' *JCEM: The Journal of Clinical Endocrinology & Metabolism*, 1 May 2013

Seaborg, E., 'Underdiagnosed & undertreated: The mysteries of genitourinary syndrome of menopause, *Endocrine News*, December 2016

Simon, J.A., Davis, S.R., et al, 'Sexual well-being after menopause: An International Menopause Society White Paper', *Climacteric,* 10 July 2018

Organisations

American College of Obstetricians and Gynecologists
acog.org

Australian Menopause Society
menopause.org.au

International Menopause Society
imsociety.org

Jean Hailes for Women's Health
jeanhailes.org.au

MJH Life Sciences
contemporaryobgyn.net

North American Menopause Society
menopause.org

Royal Australian and New Zealand College of Obstetricians
and Gynaecologists
ranzcog.edu.au

Royal College of Obstetricians and Gynaecologists
rcog.org.uk

INDEX

moisturisers 87–8, 201, 283
monoamine oxidase 62, 117
mood problems *see* mental health
moon cups 164
music 145

nails, brittleness of 291
Naltrexone 220
Naproxen 167, 172
nausea 32
negative ions 131–2
neurokinin B 53, 72
neutraceutical supplements 276
niacinamide 263–5, 268, 282
night sweats 52
nitrogen 189
NKB 53, 72
non-breast breast pain 197
non-cyclical breast pain 197
non-haem iron 175
non-steroidal anti-inflammatory drugs
    167–8
noradrenaline 117, 133
North American Menopause Society 21, 39,
    41, 56–8, 62, 67, 69–70, 90
the nose 286–7
NT-814 23
Nurses' Health Study 11, 178
nutrition *see* diet

obesity 22, 160, 192, 206, 209, 218, 224–5
obstructive sleep apnoea 160
octinoxate 259
octylmethoxycinnamate 259
oestradiol 28, 36, 42, 135
oestriol 42–3
oestrogen 28, 34, 38, 42–4, 49, 52, 80–1,
    95, 102–3, 108, 117, 151, 165, 167,
    200–1, 204, 230–1, 274, 283
oestrogen receptors 76, 98, 116
oestrogen therapy 9–11, 25–7
    see also hormone replacement therapy
oestrone (E1) 42–3
omega-3 fatty acids 129, 246–7
oral contraceptives 34–5
oral HRT 27, 31
orexin A 151
orexin antagonists 156

orexins 151
orgasm 78, 105
Orlistat 220
Ospemifeme 89
osteoporosis 10, 15, 30, 43, 194–6
ovarian cancer 7, 173
ovaries 7, 42, 48–9, 165
'overactive bladder' 99
oxybenzone 258–9
Oxybutynin 63, 84
oxygen 189
oxytocin 78

pain 191–3
pain-killers 89
pap tests 173
parabens 87, 95
parents, caring for 119
Paroxetine 62, 134
partners, advice for 297–9
passionflower 128
patches 27, 103
pedicures 201
peels 268, 272–3, 281
peer review process 6
pellets 38
pelvic floor muscles, strengthening of 90,
    101–2, 111
pelvic organ prolapse 110–13
PENN-5 staging system 48
Penn Ovarian Aging Study 118
peppermint oil 185
peptides 276
perfume 93, 95
peri visceral fat 208
perimenopause 7, 26–7, 31, 34, 41–2, 44,
    46, 48–50, 164–5, 184
periods 42, 163–8, 196–7
pessaries 38, 111–12
petroleum jelly 87, 95, 291
pets 146
Pfizer 18
pharmaceutical companies 3, 10, 17–18
pharmacies 36–8
Phentermine 219
physical activity 53, 88, 121, 143, 154–5,
    182, 192, 194, 217–18, 227, 233
phytoestrogen 67

skill learning 239
the skin 4, 201, 249–83, 286–91
skin cancer 195
Skin Cancer Foundation (US) 257
skin creams 267–8
skin pigmentation 267–9
skincare products 4, 250–2, 282–3
sleep 29, 51–2, 57, 72, 86, 121, 149–61, 181–2, 237, 275
sleep apnoea 159–61
sleep deprivation 86, 121, 150–1, 205–6, 237
sleep hygiene 152–3, 155
sleeping pills 89, 155–7
small intestinal bacterial overgrowth (SIBO) 281
smiling 141–2
smoking 41, 53, 56, 160, 169, 194, 281
snacks 179–80, 209
snoring 159–60
soap 93, 95, 260
socialising 234
socioeconomic status 53
sodium laurel sulphate 260
sodium lauryl methyl isethionate 260
soft drinks 214–15
sorbitol 191
sorbolene 93
soy isoflavones 65
SPF 257
spironolactone 285
sports bras 198
sprays 27, 31
squamous cells 254
SSRIs 134
St John's wort 70, 127
steatoblepharon 291
stepping back 142–3
steroid hormones 46–7
steroids 95–6
stiffness 191
stool lubricants 188
stool softeners 187
stress 91–2, 119–20, 139, 199, 207, 281
stress incontinence 99, 105, 173
strokes 13, 61
Study of Women's Health Across the Nation (SWAN) 191

subcutaneous fat layer 253–5
sugary snacks 179–80
sun spots 267
sunlight 195, 255, 281
sunscreens 256–9, 281
'super flushers' 54
'superfoods' 236
supplements, for skin care 275–8
suprachiasmatic nucleus (SCN) 150
surfactants 260
surgery 104, 112–13, 168–70, 172–4, 226–7, 288–91
surgical menopause 7
Suvorexant 151, 156
symptoms, of menopause 12, 44, 75, 297
synapses 238
synthetic mesh 104

T3 161–2
T4 161–2
tablets 27, 29, 80
tachyphylaxis 38
Tamoxifen 7, 30, 62, 170, 199
task management 143
tau 237
tea 176, 194
testosterone 31, 38, 44–6, 48, 78, 81–5, 231–2, 241, 284, 299
tetraiodothyronine 161–2
Therapeutic Goods Administration 36–7
thermoneutral zone 53, 56
thrush 92, 96–7
thyroid disease 161–3
thyroid gland 89, 161
thyroid replacement therapy 162–3
thyroxine 161–2
Tibolone 31, 60–1, 66–7, 81, 84–5, 200
Tietze's disease 197
#TimesUp 23
tip ptosis 286
tiredness 149–51, 163, 177, 181–2, 202
tissue-selective estrogen complex (TSEC) 61–2, 200
titanium dioxide 258
tocopherol 242
Topiramate 219
Toremifene 199
TpH2 17